Tai Chi Beginning

A Complete Workout Reference for Beginners

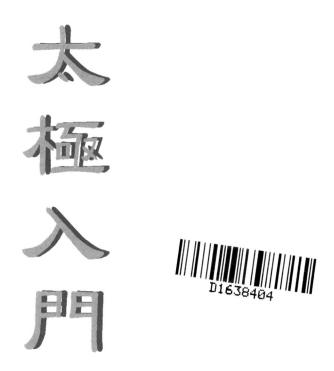

太極入門

By **Wen-Ching Wu**

The Way of the Dragon Publishing, Rhode Island, U.S.A.

Published by:

The Way of the Dragon Publishing
P. O. Box 14561
East Providence, RI 02914-0561
United States of America

Copyright © 1998, by Wen-Ching Wu

Printed in the United States of America

First Printing 1998

On Demand Edition 2017

Publisher's Cataloging-in-Publication Data

Wu, Wen-Ching, 1964-

Tai chi beginning: a complete workout reference for beginners / Wen-Ching Wu

illus.   p.   cm.

Includes bibliographical references and index.

ISBN 1-889659-03-7

1. Tai Chi Chuan. 2. Qi (Chinese philosophy). 3 Qigong. I. Breiter-Wu, Denise. II. Title.

GV504.L53   1998   786.815'5   98-60194

Table of Contents

Acknowledgments

Thank you to Sarah Alexander, Frank Whitsitt-Lynch, and Gail Whitsitt-Lynch, for proof reading the manuscript and for contributing valuable suggestions. Our greatest appreciation to all of our friends and students who have contributed to this book indirectly through their questions and encouragement over the years.

Dedication

To my parents, and my teachers Master Liang, Shou-Yu, Professor Wang, Ju-Rong, and Dr. Wu, Cheng-De for their unconditional love, knowledge, and guidance.

Warning-Disclaimer

The exercises in this book may be too mentally and physically demanding for some people. Readers should use their own discretion and consult their doctor before engaging in these exercises. The author and the publisher shall have neither liability nor responsibility to any person or entity with respect to any loss or damage caused, or alleged to be caused, directly or indirectly by reading or following the instructions in this book.

Introduction

Taijiquan (Tai Chi Chuan) is a series of graceful movements directed with focused intention that enhances a smooth flow of qi (energy) in the body. This intention assists in balancing the qi in the body while training the mind to attain a better focus. Your desire to take control of your health and well-being with Taijiquan will assist you in realizing the connectedness of your mind, body, and qi. With the balanced development of the mind, body and qi in your Taijiquan practice, you can attain better health and well-being.

The theory in Taijiquan is based on the philosophy of Yin-Yang. It is a philosophy of dynamic balance; opposition, yet interdependence; and transformation. Everything can be classified and explained with the Yin-Yang philosophy — the computer's binary numbers, night and day, female and male, up and down, etc.

In the thousands of years since the Yin-Yang philosophy was formulated, many different symbols have been drawn to represent the philosophy. The symbol on the following page is a typical representation. This symbol is referred to as a Taiji (Tai Chi) Symbol from which, Taijiquan borrowed its name. (The third syllable, *quan (chuan)* means *fist* or *style of martial arts*.)

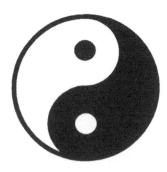

Taiji Symbol

In the Taiji Symbol, the big circle on the outside represents the entire universe. The dark part of the symbol represents yin, and the white part represents yang. The curvature between the yin and the yang represents the opposing, yet interdependent nature of yin and yang. The tear drop shapes represent the decreasing and increasing, as well as, the transformation of yin into yang and yang into yin. The smaller white or black dot within the tear drop shape represents the inherent yin or yang within yang or yin. That is yin and yang are not absolute; within yin, there is yang; and within yang, there is yin; and each can be further divided into yin and yang.

The Yin-Yang philosophy is an attempt to explain how nature works. It is also a philosophy that emphasizes balance and the wisdom of being natural. Being natural doesn't mean not doing anything. It means making choices that go along with the natural patterns. Being natural doesn't mean that one can't make conscious decisions or choices. As we go through life, we are faced with choices everyday. Whether we choose to make the choice or not, is still making a choice. When we make decisions in accordance with nature, and truly allow that which is in accordance with nature to be, we will be in a state of balance with ourselves, as well as, with others and our environment.

Taijiquan (Tai Chi Chuan) is an exercise based on returning the body to a natural state. It is both a physical exercise and an internal exercise. It is a healing/martial art that combines martial arts movements with qi circulation, breathing, and stretching techniques.

The physical part of Taijiquan is a set of movements designed to exercise every bone, muscle, joint, and ligament in the body. There are forward, backward, sideways, upward, and downward movements. At the completion of the routine, you will have exercised every part of your body from your head down to your toes, including your internal organs.

The Taijiquan movements train the individual to achieve the highest physical efficiency and potential through a series of condensing and extending movements, along with physically symmetrical movements. The condensing and extending, and physically symmetrical movements allow the body to achieve a dynamic energy equilibrium. These movements also train the different parts of the body to become an integrated series of *pumps*. Instead of relying on the heart to pump the blood and energy around, the entire body is involved in Taijiquan practice.

This total body exercise includes the ribs, spine, and internal organs. The gentle movements loosen the muscles around the spine and ribs, as well as, *massages* the internal organs. Realizing that most major illnesses are caused by problems associated with the internal organs, one of the objectives in Taijiquan practice is to directly or indirectly *massage* the internal organs. Taijiquan's internal organ massage can stimulate the flow of blood and energy to reduce stagnation and provide better blood and energy circulation to and from the lungs.

The slow movements of Taijiquan allow the body to move with less tension than fast pace movements, which require quick muscle contractions. The slow movements also allow the lungs to be more relaxed and to increase the intake of oxygen.

The constant condensing and expanding movements work on stretching the muscles and allow the joints to open up for better energy circulation. Since muscles only contract, the part of the body that is being stretched is *relaxed* through the gentle contraction of muscles in the other parts of the body.

For example, in a forward push, when the wrist settles and the fingers extend from a naturally coiled position, the palm is being stretched *open*. Keep in mind that Taijiquan is a continuous flow of movement from one posture to the next, with no part of the body remaining static. Different parts of the body are being stretched as you go through the routine.

The internal training in Taijiquan is the qi (energy) cultivation. Qi is the intrinsic substance within all things in the universe, including the human body. The internal energy practice can assist in the healing of illness, by building the qi to counteract the pathogenic influences and to regulate the balance of qi, thereby returning the body to a normal physiological state.

In Taijiquan practice, energy cultivation can be accomplished through the conscious regulation of the body movements. By placing your intention on your movements, qi will be lead by your mind to the specific areas of your intention. For example, when your mind is placed on the symmetrical movements, you put the body in a position that allows for energetic balance. That is, use physical symmetry to attain energetic balance.

The focus on qi (energy) in Taijiquan was used for the purpose of increasing the internal strength of the physical body for combat. The same techniques that were capable of developing internal power for combat, have also been proven to be effective as life prolonging, healing and rejuvenating exercises. These health benefits are the primary contributions that have led to the popularity of Taijiquan today.

In today's world, people are often too busy to be concerned about their health, until their health becomes a problem. Luckily modern medicine has a cure for many common diseases. Unfortunately, there are some that are still incurable. Often times the root of an illness is not corrected and the illness reoccurs or manifests itself in other forms. The value of Taijiquan is in its potential to strengthen and repair the physical and energetic body, which in turn has the potential to prevent and cure diseases.

With the regular practice of Taijiquan, you can help keep blood and energy circulation smooth in the entire body, and prevent disease. Traditional Chinese Medicine places prevention, correcting a potential problem before any physical manifestation occurs, as the highest regard. If a problem already exists, it can be regulated through the regular practice of Taijiquan, before it causes any major damage. The slow non-jarring, integrated movements of Taijiquan are an excellent recovery exercise after suffering from an illness, to regain health.

Taijiquan can also help release tension created by a hard day at work. Mental and energetic tension is released from the head and other areas where energy stagnates. Modern science has documented that each section of our brain does a specialized set of tasks. Over the course of the day, week, month, or year, one section of the brain may be overstimulated. This overstimulation often creates excess tension that is hard to dissipate from the head. When this happens, people may not be able to think as clearly, get irritated easily, get headaches.... Prolonged disharmony or energy imbalance in the body will increase disease (dis-ease), a lack of ease. Taijiquan practice is a method of living with ease and preventing disease.

Taijiquan redistributes energy in the body, by leading excess energy from tense areas to regain balance. Performing Taijiquan early in the morning clears the mind, balances your emotions, and prepares one to tackle the tasks of the day. That is one of the reasons, to the amazement of many foreign visitors to China, that millions of Chinese practice Taijiquan in the park every morning before work.

Beside practicing Taijiquan regularly, proper hygiene, diet, and maintaining a positive mental attitude, are also important for staying healthy. When one practices Taijiquan, yet constantly abuses one's body with unhealthy habits, one renders one's practice ineffective. Life is precious and hard to come by, one should not waste this opportunity.

Today, we are thankful for medical advances in treating many life threatening illnesses. However, this technology can't keep us healthy and it doesn't relinquish our responsibility for our own well-being. We can rely on doctors for checkups and to give us suggestions for staying healthy, but we can't rely on them to keep us healthy. We are ultimately responsible for our own well-being. By taking an active role in acquiring better health, and with consistent practice, you will be able to gain the highest benefits from your Taijiquan practice.

Your interest in this book is an indication of your desire to begin or continue your search for greater well-being. It is our hope that this book will be instrumental in sparking a desire to continue to learn and benefit from the practice of Taijiquan.

Tai Chi Beginning Contents

This book is designed as a training reference specifically for beginners. It focuses on body mechanics and energy development which will provide health and healing benefits, as well as, build a good foundation for anyone interested in Taijiquan as a martial art. Whether you are interested in Taijiquan for health or for martial arts, proper body mechanics and an energetic foundation are essential to achieve the best possible benefits and results in your practice.

This book consists of three chapters. Chapter 1 includes a description of simple warm up exercises to prepare the body for movement. It also includes a simple spinal exercise to relax the muscles around the spine allowing a smooth flow of movement through the torso. Chapter 2 includes a simple 10 minute Taiji Qigong exercise to assist you in balancing your qi (energy). This exercise will help you benefit from your Taijiquan practice, by developing your sensitivity to your qi; and to begin the coordination of your body with your mind, breathing, and qi.

For people that have never felt a manifestation of their qi, it is an enlightening experience to feel your qi for the first time. In our classroom and in our workshops, 90% or more of the participants are able to feel their qi, the first time they practice this simple qigong exercise. Once you have felt your qi, you will have more confidence in your Taijiquan practice.

Chapter 3 is the main part of this book. It consists of the 24 Posture Taijiquan (Tai Chi Chuan). It is also known as Simplified Taijiquan. Explanations of the movement mechanics, notes, and the layout are all carefully planned to ensure ease of learning.

Chapter 1:

Warm Up & Spinal Exercise

1.1. Warm Up

When doing any type of exercise, it is always advisable to do some warm up exercises and stretching. It is not only important to get your physical body ready, but your mind must also be ready to exercise. This is especially true for Taijiquan, since the intent of your mind leads the movements of your body.

There are nine areas that you need to pay attention to when warming up for any exercise (Figure 1-1). They are the wrist area (including your hand joints), the elbows, the shoulders, the ankles (including your foot and toe joints), the knees, the hips, and the three sections of your spine — the lumbar, the thoracic, and the cervical vertebra.

The *Tai Chi Beginning Workout* video has a warm up routine that works on the nine major areas in the body. This set of exercises can also be done in addition to your other stretching/warm up exercises.

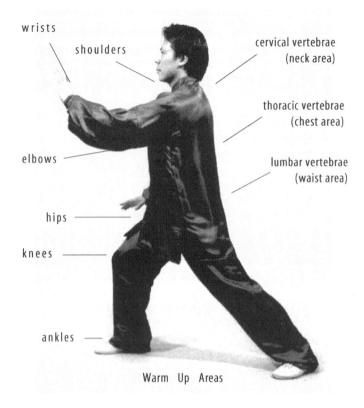

wrists
shoulders
cervical vertebrae
(neck area)
thoracic vertebrae
(chest area)
lumbar vertebrae
(waist area)
elbows
hips
knees
ankles

Warm Up Areas

Suggested warm up exercise:

Step 1. Stand with your feet shoulder width apart (use this stance for steps 1 to 6). Gently shake your wrists and fingers. Do 10 to 20 times.

Step 2. Extend the shaking movement up to your elbows so that the entire arm is shaking. Do 10 to 20 times.

Step 3. Relax your arms. Bounce your upper body up and down, by bending your knees slightly then straightening them continuously. Keep your upper body as loose as possible. This will gently move your shoulders up and down as you bounce with your legs. Do 10 to 20 times.

Step 4. Relax your arms. Turn your waist and hips from side to side. Allow your arms to also swing from side to side as your waist and hips turn. Do 10 to 20 times.

Step 5. Bring both arms over your head and circle both arms in front of your body. When circling your arms, reach your arms up as high as you are comfortable with, and lower your arms down as low as you are comfortable with, by bending from your waist. Do 10 to 20 times then reverse directions 10 to 20 times.

Step 6. Place your hands on your waist and move your waist in a circular pattern Make as big a circle as you are comfortable with. Do 10 to 20 times, then reverse directions.

Step 7. Bring your feet together and bend your knees as low as you are comfortable with. Next, place your hands gently on top of your knees.

Gently move your knees in a circular pattern. Make as big a circle as you are comfortable with. Do 10 to 20 times, then reverse directions 10 to 20 times.

Step 8. Stand up, place your hands on your waist, and extend your right foot slightly behind you. Most of your weight should be on your left foot.

Gently move your ankle in a circular pattern. Make as big a circle as you are comfortable with. Do 10 to 20 times, then reverse directions.

Step 9. Repeat Step 8 with your left foot by shifting your weight onto your right foot and placing your left foot slightly behind you.

Step 10. Bring your feet together. Interlock both hands and reach up over your head with your palms facing up.

Then turn your body as far as you are comfortable with to one side, back to the center, then to the other side with your arms still over head. Again, bring your body back to the center and repeat the turning one more time.

Next, bend your body sideways from your waist with your arms over your head. Bring your body back to the center and bend your body to the other side. Again, bring your body back to the center and bend your body from side to side.

Step 11. Repeat Step 10.

Step 12. Stand with your feet about two shoulder widths apart with your feet turned out slightly. Squat down on one leg as low as you can. Make sure your knee and foot are pointing in the same direction, while keeping the other leg straight. Hold this position for 10 to 20 seconds then change sides and hold for 10 to 20 seconds.

Step 13. Repeat Step 12, except this time, the foot of the straight leg points up.

Step 14. Sit down on the floor with your feet together and legs straight. Straighten your back and lean forward as far as you can, while reaching forward with your hands. Hold this position for 10 to 20 seconds.

Relax and sit back up, then reach forward again and hold for 10 to 20 seconds.

Step 15. Move your feet apart as far as you can. Again, straighten your back and lean forward as far as you can, while reaching forward with your hands. Hold this position for 10 to 20 seconds.

Relax and sit back up, then reach forward again and hold for 10 to 20 seconds.

Step 16. Reach over your head with one arm towards your opposite foot. Hold this position for 10 to 20 seconds, then change sides and hold for 10 to 20 seconds.

1.2. Spinal Exercise

The movement or the lack of movement of the spine affects the entire body including the organs. Moving the spine can enhance the flow of qi in your body. It is easier to move the arms and legs, than it is to gain control of the torso movements. Being able to move the torso, including the spine, hips, and waist, will increase the fluidity of your Taijiquan movements and improve the flow of qi in your body.

Below we will introduce a simple method that will help train your ability to move your torso. This spinal exercise is a simplified version to help you gain better control of your spinal movements.

Movement:

Step 1. Stand with your feet shoulder width apart with your knees slightly bent.

Step 2. Gently place one hand on your abdomen and the other hand on the small of your back, front palm faces in and back palm faces out (Figure 1-1).

Loosen the joints between your hips and your lumbar vertebra, by gently making horizontal circles with your waist and hips (Figure 1-2). Repeat 10 times.

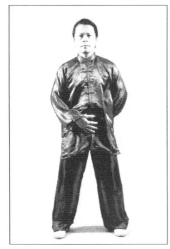

Figure 1-1

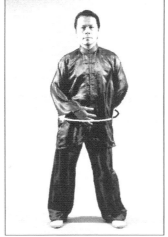

Figure 1-2

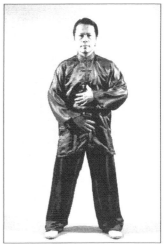

Figure 1-3

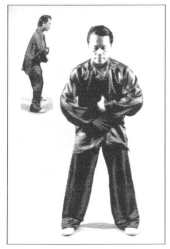

Figure 1-4

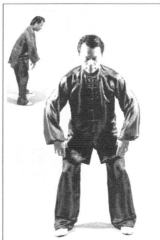

Figure 1-5

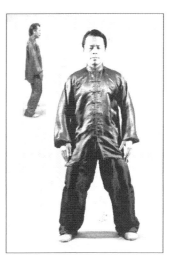

Figure 1-6

Step 3. Keep your hands in the same place and reverse the circular movement. Repeat 10 times.

Step 4. Keep your front hand on your abdomen and gently place your other hand over your solar plexus area. Roll your body in a wavelike motion from your hips up to your mid spine (Figures 1-3 and 1-4). Repeat 10 times.

Step 5. Relax your arms to your sides. Roll your body in a wavelike motion as in Step 4, except allow the wavelike motion to continue all the way up to your head (Figures 1-5 and 1-6).

The movement can be as big or as small as you are comfortable with. Repeat 10 times.

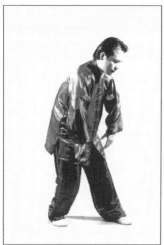 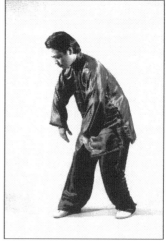

Figure 1-7   Figure 1-8

Step 6. Turn your feet and body slightly to one side and repeat Step 5 (Figure 1-7).

Step 7. Turn your feet and body to the other side and repeat Step 5 (Figure 1-8).

Notes:

1. Pay attention to the specific area being worked on. With practice you will be able to move your torso in any direction with ease.

2. It is not critical that you move your spine exactly as shown in the exercise, as long as, you are able to move your spine effortlessly in any possible direction.

Chapter 2:

Feel the Qi

2.1. The Energy Concept

As we emerge from the space age and realize the similarities between Quantum Physics and ancient Eastern philosophy, many of the ancient Eastern practices are being reevaluated. The resurgence of Eastern practices are spreading rapidly to the West. As their popularity grows, so are the mysteries and intrigues that come along with these practices. Many of these ancient ways can't be proven with Western scientific reasoning, yet they have lasted through the millenniums, helping, and guiding our ancestors. One of the most influential ancient practices involves the use of acupuncture to balance *qi*, an intrinsic energetic substance. Millions of people have benefited from acupuncture for healing illness, strengthening the body, and preventing illness.

Generally speaking, qi is the intrinsic substance that makes up the cosmos, and produces all things through its movement. Qi is the medium between and within all material substances. We are all immersed in it. The physiological definition of qi in Traditional Chinese Medicine is the *intrinsic substance* that flows in the human body and is the impelling force for all living activities. It is not visible to the ordinary eye. However, it can be felt by most people.

19

Qi, like the current in an electric wire, is not visible like physical materials. But, it can manifest in many ways, such as, a magnetic force, warmth, coolness, and/or a tingling sensation. Qi in our body includes the energy derived from air, food, and water, as well as, the innate energy source we inherit from our parents. The existence of qi is felt indirectly and manifests as a result of the human body's interactions within its integral parts and with the environment.

Every set of qigong (the study or attainment of qi) involves the mind, body postures and movements, breathing, and/or vocalization. People use different approaches in their qigong practices for attaining a variety of goals. Healers and people that take an active role in their health use qigong for healing and preventing illness. Martial artists use qigong for developing incredible strength and abilities. Others practice qigong to help integrate the physical body with the *innerself* and to develop a higher awareness of being.

Under normal conditions, the human body is in an energetically balanced state that is capable of maintaining its physiological functions and can adapt to changes in the environment. When the pathogenic influences, including stress, are above and beyond the normal functioning of the body, and the body is unable to adjust; the normal physiological functions will be destroyed. This will create energetic obstructions and result in illness. That is to say, the occurrence of illness is not only strongly related to pathogenic influences; it is also strongly dependent on the adaptability of the human body to our changing environment.

If qi in the human body is strong, then it will be difficult for the pathogenic influences to adversely affect the body. Even if the pathogenic influences do attack the body, the abundance of qi will increase the immunity of the body and prevent disease from occurring. Only when qi is weak or deficient, will the pathogenic influences be able to cause irregularities in the physiological systems, resulting in dis-ease or illness.

The way traditional Chinese medical doctors, acupuncturists, and other healers remove the physical manifestation of an illness is by acupuncture treatments, prescribing drugs, herbs, or nutritional supplements. In serious cases, surgery may have to be performed to prevent further damage. External assistance is not a permanent solution to problems associated with energetic imbalance. Without a life-style change, after the external assistance has stopped, the individual's body may still not have a natural response to prevent the illness from reoccurring.

One life-style change includes working on maintaining the balance and building of energy within the body. By practicing qigong and/or Taijiquan regularly, the natural response to establish an energetic balance within the body can be achieved and strengthened. This is the key to preventing illness from remanifesting in a similar or other forms

After the former U.S. President, Richard Nixon, visited China in the 1970's and witnessed open heart surgery with the application of acupuncture in place of general anesthesia, the interest in acupuncture and qi escalated at an exponential rate in the U.S. Today there are acupuncturists all over the world helping to heal people with all types of illnesses. As the popularity of acupuncture grew, so did the self-healing counterpart of this energetic system — the practice of Taijiquan and qigong.

Another boost to the popularity of the ancient Chinese ways was the PBS show on *Healing and the Mind* presented by Bill Moyers. In the segment on qi filmed in China, Bill Moyers showed Qigong healers using acupuncture, massage, and emitting qi to heal patients. He also showed people practicing Taijiquan and qigong in the park for healing and for building qi.

For a more complete explanation about qigong and the types of qigong available please refer to *Qigong Empowerment* by Master Shou-Yu Liang and Wen-Ching Wu.

2.2. Taiji (Tai Chi) Qigong

This exercise includes the combined essence of Taijiquan and qigong. It is called Taiji Qigong. It can be practiced by itself or with Taijiquan routines. The practice of Taiji Qigong can elevate sluggish energy, due to the excessive demands of daily activities, providing more energy to tackle our tasks. It can also help reduce stress and retain balance for a more relaxing evening and rest.

Taiji Qigong is very versatile in its practice. It can be practiced while standing or sitting, in work clothes or casual clothes, at home or at work, indoors or outdoors; requiring only the space equal to the span of your arms. After practicing this 10 Minute Taiji Qigong, you will feel energized, refreshed, more relaxed and alert. This can significantly improve your health and performance in anything you do.

Taiji Qigong is an effective energetic health exercise based on the same theories as in Traditional Chinese Medicine and Acupuncture. Since the arms and legs are the outer connections of the qi channels that link to the internal organs, moving the arms in specific patterns, can enhance the flow of qi in these energy pathways and help regain energetic balance.

This exercise consists of 6 simple, but powerful energy balancing and strengthening movements. By following the specific movements and breathing patterns, and paying attention to your movements, you will generate and bring about a stronger circulation of qi in your body. The simple arm movements coordinated with your breathing and mind, will also prepare you for the more challenging Taijiquan routine to follow.

After completing this simple qigong set, bring your palms next to each other, but without touching them. You may feel that your palms are warm, cool, and/or tingling. You may also feel a magnetic repulsion feeling between your palms, as if you had two of magnets of the same poles repelling each other. All of these sensations are an indication of the presence and heighten flow of qi. Below is the description for the 6 piece Taiji Qigong exercise. In a workout session, it is recommended that you repeat each piece of the exercise, six times.

Preparation

Start from a standing position, place your hands with your palms facing down, in front of your body (Figure 2-1). Your elbows should be bent slightly, just enough for your palms to face down when you settle your wrist and extend your fingers to point forward.

The level of your hands is about three inches below your navel, at your center of gravity and one of your main energy centers, known as the *dantian*.

The distance between your hands and the centerline of your body creates an equilateral triangle. We will refer to this posture as the Preparation posture, and we will be referring to the *dantian* as a reference place for your arm movements.

First Piece

Movements: (Figures 2-2 to 2-4)

Step 1. From the Preparation, allow your fingers to point down at an angle as you rotate your hands to face each other (Figure 2-2).

Then raise your hands up to shoulder level. As your hands reach shoulder level, rotate your palms until they are facing down (Figure 2-3).

Step 2. Pull your hands in slightly and lower your hands back down to the Preparation posture (Figure 2-4).

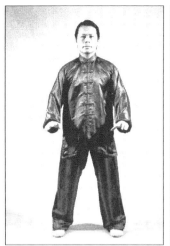

Figure 2-1

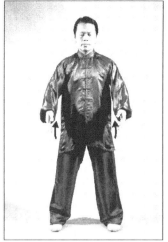

Figure 2-2

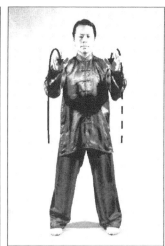

Figure 2-3

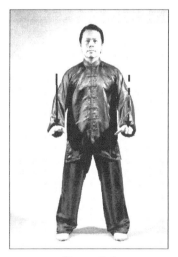

Figure 2-4

Step 3. Repeat Steps 2 and 3, a total of six times.

Notes:

1. Keep your fingers naturally coiled in when raising your hands. Settle your wrists slightly as you lower your hands.

2. The movement of your arms is like a whip with your hands moving in an oval path. To keep your hands in an oval path, you will have to move your elbows like the handle of a whip and the hands like the tip of the whip.

3. By bending your elbows right before your hands reach shoulder level, and continuing to raise your hands up to shoulder level,

will create a wave like movement. The wave like movement also allows your shoulders to be more relaxed during the exercise which helps achieve a smoother energy flow through and from your torso.

4. The breathing pattern is to inhale while raising your hands up to shoulder level, and to exhale while lowering your hands back to the starting position. In the remaining pieces, the requirements for the movements of your wrists, palms, and fingers will be similar to the first piece.

5. This is the commencing piece that brings your mind back to your body, especially to your *dantian*, your energy center. As you become smoother with your movements and breathing, gradually use more and more of your abdomen to assist you in all your movements and breathing.

Second Piece

Movements: (Figures 2-5 to 2-9)

Step 1. From the Preparation posture, cross your arms and rotate your palms to face up in front of your abdomen (Figure 2-5). Then with your arms crossed, raise both arms in front of your body (Figure 2-6).

Step 2. When your hands reach your head level, rotate your hands to face out then down, as you lower your arms down (Figure 2-7).

Continue to lower your arms until they reach your abdomen. Then, again cross your arms and rotate your palms to face up in front of your abdomen (Figures 2-8 and 2-9).

Step 3. Repeat Steps 1 and 2, a total of six times.

Notes:

1. Similar to the whip example given in the First Piece; in the Second Piece, allow your elbows to drop slightly before lowering your hands. The visualization for this movement implies getting rid of impurities and stress from the body.

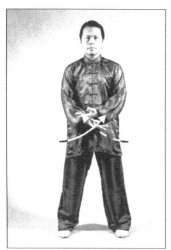

Figure 2-5

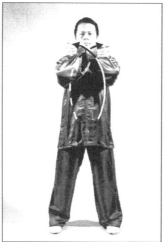

Figure 2-6

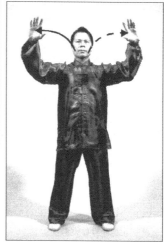

Figure 2-7

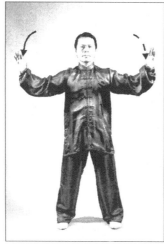

Figure 2-8

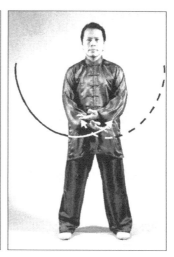

Figure 2-9

2. The breathing pattern is to inhale while raising your arms up to your head level, and to exhale while lowering your hands down to your sides. Settle your wrist and extend your fingers slightly at the completion of your exhalation.

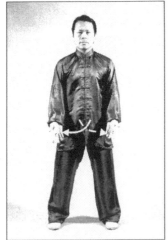
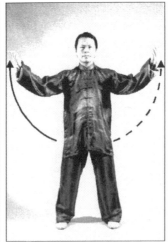
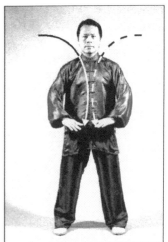

| Figure 2-10 | Figure 2-11 | Figure 2-12 |

Third Piece

Movements: (Figures 2-10 to 2-12)

Step 1. After completing the Second Piece, with your palms facing up at your abdomen, lower your palms down, turning your palms to face forward (Figure 2-10).

Then rotate your hands to face palm up as you raise your arms up to your head level (Figure 2-11).

Step 2. Bend your elbows so that your palms are facing down and begin lowering your hands down in front of your body to your abdomen level (Figure 2-12).

Step 3. Continue lowering your arms, rotate your palms to face out as in Step 1, and repeat the Third piece, a total of six times.

Notes:

1. When lowering your hands down, keep your index fingers and thumbs of both hands next to each other, but not touching, forming a triangle as you lower your hands.

The Third Piece is the reverse of the Second Piece. The visualization for this movement resembles the gathering of the *pure essence* from the universe to nourish your body.

2. Inhale, as you raise your hands up over your head. Exhale, as you lower your hands down in front of your body.

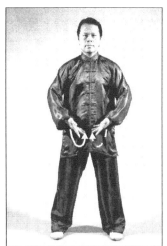

Figure 2-13

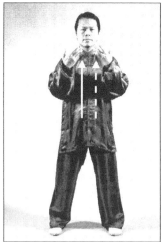

Figure 2-14

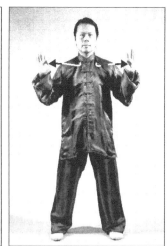

Figure 2-15

Fourth Piece

Movements: (Figures 2-13 to 2-19)

Step 1. At the completion of the third piece, when your hands have reached your abdomen, rotate your palms to face up (Figure 2-13).

Raise your arms up in front of your body. As your hands reach your chest level, drop your elbows, and rotate your hands so your palms face forward (Figures 2-14 and 2-15).

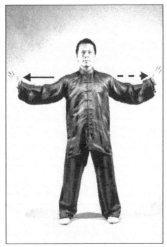 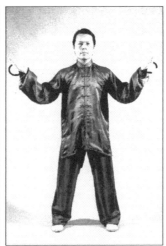 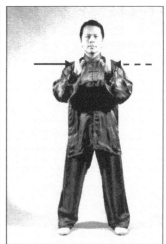

Figure 2-16   Figure 2-17   Figure 2-18

Step 2. Continue to rotate your palms until they are facing away
from your sides as you extend and push your palms out to
your sides (Figure 2-16).

Step 3. Next, bend your elbows and rotate your hands to face
each other, and pull your hands back towards the center
of your body (Figures 2-17 and 2-18).

Then fold your forearms and palms to face down, and
lower both hands down to your *dantian* level (Figure 2-
19).

Step 4. To repeat, again rotate your hands so your palms face up
and raise them up towards your chest and repeat the
Fourth Piece, a total of six times.

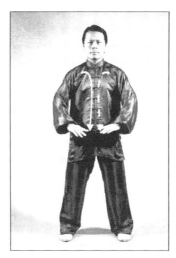

Figure 2-19

Notes:

1. When extending your arms to the side, do not extend your arms too far back and lock your shoulder blades.

2. The Fourth Piece requires two inhalations and two exhalations to complete. Inhale when you raise your hands up to your chest level and begin to rotate your palms facing forward. Exhale, when you extend your arms to the sides. Then, again inhale, when you pull your hands back towards your chest. And, exhale again, as you rotate your palms to face down and push your hands down to your *dantian* level.

3. The visualization for the movement of this piece, as well as, the Fifth Piece resembles the action of pushing unwanted things away, and bringing pleasant things back towards your body.

   It is as though you are gathering *pure essence* during the inhalation and expanding your energy to form a strong guardian layer *(guardian-qi)* around your body to fend off pathogenic influences.

29

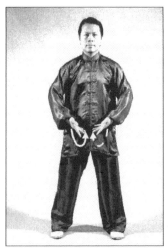
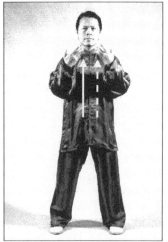
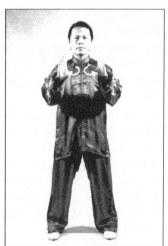

| Figure 2-20 | Figure 2-21 | Figure 2-22 |

Fifth Piece

Movements: (Figures 2-20 to 2-26)

Step 1. At the completion of the Fourth Piece, when your hands have reached your abdomen, again rotate your hands so your palms face up (Figure 2-20).

Raise your palms up in front of your body. As your hands reach your chest level, drop your elbows, and rotate your hands so your palms face forward (Figures 2-21 and 2-22).

Step 2. Next, extend and push forward with your palms (Figure 2-23).

Step 3. Next, bend your elbows and rotate your hands so your palms face in, and pull your hands back towards your body (Figures 2-24 and 2-25).

Then fold your forearms and palms to face down, and lower both hands down to your dantian level (Figure 2-26).

Step 4. To repeat, again rotate your hands so your palms face up. Raise them up towards your chest, and repeat the Fifth Piece, a total of six times.

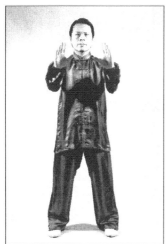

Figure 2-23

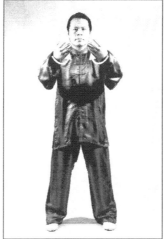

Figure 2-24

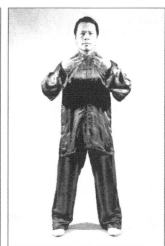

Figure 2-25

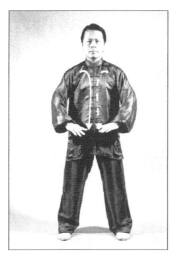

Figure 2-26

Notes:

1. The Fifth Piece also requires two inhalations and two exhalations to complete. Inhale, when you raise your hands up to your chest level and begin to rotate your palms to face forward. Exhale, when you extend your arms forward. Then, again inhale, when you pull your hands back towards your chest. And, exhale again, as you rotate your palms to face down and push your hands down to your *dantian* level.

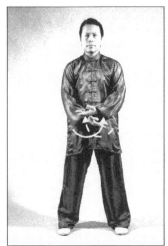 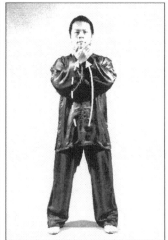 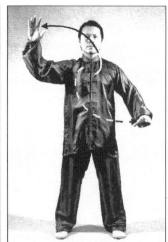

Figure 2-27   Figure 2-28   Figure 2-29

Sixth Piece

Movements: (Figures 2-27 to 2-31)

Step 1. At the completion of the Fifth Piece, again rotate your hands so your palms face up (Figure 2-27). Then, cross your forearms on top of each other as you raise both hands up to your throat level (Figure 2-28).

Next, extend your right hand up to the right upper corner and extend the left hand to the left lower corner (Figure 2-29).

Step 2. Bring your hands back to your throat level and cross your forearms (Figure 2-30).

Next, extend your left hand up to the left upper corner and extend the right hand to the right lower corner (Figure 2-31).

Step 3. Again, cross your forearms in front of your throat and repeat the up and down extension of your arms from one side to the next. Do a total of six times each side.

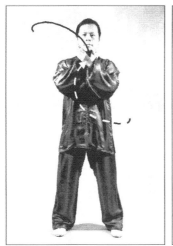 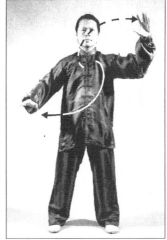

Figure 2-30   Figure 2-31

Notes:

1. Don't be overly concerned with which arm crosses in the front or the back. Be natural with the way your arms cross.

   Also, it doesn't make any difference which hand extends up first. Simply do an even number of times on each side.

2. The Sixth Piece resembles a bird shaking water off its wet feathers. At the completion of your arm extension, keep your elbows slightly bent. The upper hand should be facing forward and the lower hand facing down.

3. The Sixth Piece also requires two inhalations and two exhalations to complete. Inhale, when your arms are crossing. Exhale, when you extend your arms.

Closing

Movements: (Figures 2-32 to 2-35)

Step 1. To finish this Taiji Qigong exercise, cross your hands, palms facing in, in front of your throat (Figure 2-32).

Step 2. Rotate both palms to face down and separate your hands until they are a shoulder width apart (Figures 2-33 and 2-34).

Step 3. Then bend both elbows and lower both hands down to your *dantian* level, as in the Preparation posture (Figure 2-35).

Notes:

1. Inhale, when you cross your hands and separate your hands. Exhale, when you lower your hands.

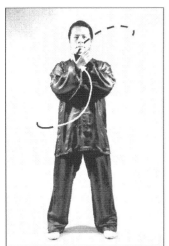

Figure 2-32

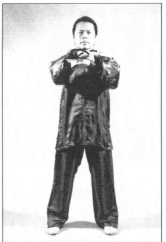

Figure 2-33

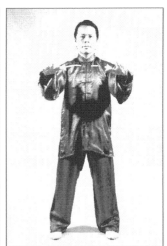

Figure 2-34

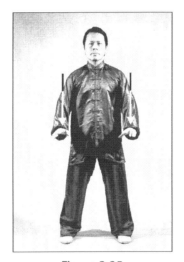

Figure 2-35

Emitting and Sensing Your Qi

Step 1. Rotate your palms until they are facing each other in front of your abdomen. Next, bring your palms close to each other without touching. Then pull them away from each other. Repeat as many time as you like (Figures 2-36 and 2-37)

When your palms are moving towards each other, gently flex your palm and extend your fingers. Return your palms to a naturally coiled position as you pull your palms apart.

Pay attention to the warmth, tingling, and/or magnetic repulsion sensations between your palms.

Step 2. Point the fingers of your right hand towards your left palm, without touching, and brush your fingers up and down the length of your left palm (Figure 2-38).

Pay attention to the qi projected from your fingers as it tickles your left palm.

Step 3. Draw circles in the air over your left palm and pay attention to the qi projected from your fingers (Figure 2-39).

Step 4. Repeat Steps 2 and 3 by projecting qi from the fingers of your left hand and sensing it with your right palm.

General Notes:

1. Everyone has qi. Since the human body has qi, bioelectrical activity, it can generate a *field* — a space within which magnetic or electrical lines of force are active. Most people are able to feel this field after proper qigong training. Some may even be able to see the light or aura of this field.

2. Breathing is a process that we often take for granted. We were never taught how to breathe, it simply came naturally when we were born. However, as we get older, partly due to a weakening and/or lack of exercise of the primary muscles associated with breathing, we begin to lose the full capacity of our lungs. Older individuals often find themselves breathing shallower and at a faster pace, than when they were younger. This could be due to the loss of efficiency of the intercostal (rib) muscles and the diaphragm.

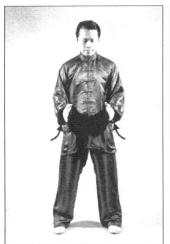

Figure 2-36

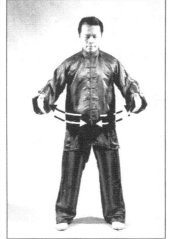

Figure 2-37

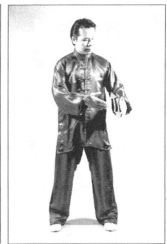

Figure 2-38

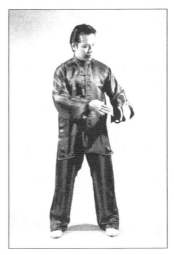

Figure 2-39

The mechanics of breathing have two aspects: inhalation and exhalation. To inhale, the atmospheric pressure in the lungs must be lower than the atmospheric pressure of the environment. During inhalation, the pressure in the lungs is reduced by lung expansion. This increases the volume of the lungs, thereby reducing the pressure in the lungs and allowing the higher pressured air from the outside to enter the lungs. To increase the volume of the lungs, the diaphragm and intercostal muscles contract.

Exhalation usually happens naturally by relaxing the contracted diaphragm and intercostal muscles. The relaxation of the intercostal muscles releases the elastic-like rib cage and pushes the air out of the lungs.

Chapter 3:

Simplified Tai Chi Chuan

3.1. Basic Concepts

Traditional Taijiquan (Tai Chi Chuan) routines have been around for a long time. There are several legends about the creation of Taijiquan. One such legend believes that in the 12th or 14th century B.C., a Daoist (Taoist) priest, named Zhang San-Feng created Taijiquan after observing a fight between a crane and a snake.

Others believe that the movements which combine the energy circulation in Taijiquan originated with Chen Wang-Ting in the later part of the 1600's. Many believe that Chen Wang-Ting combined the *Martial Classics in Thirty-Two Postures* with the *Daoist Yellow Court Classic* to become what is known as Taijiquan today.

However, the energy circulation principle in Taijiquan practice can be traced back much further than Zhang San-Feng or Chen Wang-Ting. It is a theory based on the ancient Yin-Yang philosophy, a philosophy of the interdependent nature of all things in the universe. This philosophy can be traced back to the early part of Chinese civilization (5000 years ago) to the Book of Changes (Yijing or I Ching).

Today, there are several different styles of Taijiquan available. Within each of the various styles are many different routines and training methods, from the most basic to the more advanced. The major styles available today include: Chen, Yang, Wú, Wu, and Sun Styles.

The routine presented in this manual is the 24 Posture Tai Chi Chuan, also referred to as Simplified Tai Chi Chuan. It is derived from the Traditional Yang Style Taijiquan routine. It was compiled in China in 1956 by the Taijiquan masters, in an effort to standardize and simplify Taijiquan for use as a beginners' routine and as a health promoting exercise. Many of the more involved and repeated movements were deleted from the traditional routine for ease of learning and practicing. The routine starts off with very simple movements and gradually becomes more complicated. It has both left and right sides for many of the postures, in contrast to the traditional long routine, which has many one sided postures.

This routine consists of 20 different postures. Three of the more involved postures are done on both sides, and are referred to as the left or right side of that posture. One of the postures repeats itself, making a total of 24 postures, thereby, the name 24 Posture Taijiquan. It is an excellent introduction routine to Taijiquan practice.

Regardless of which Taijiquan routine you practice, they all emphasize proper body mechanics to promote the best possible energy development, flow, and balance. On the following pages are some notes and illustrations to point out some of the basic requirements to keep in mind when you practice Taijiquan. They include: 1) The symmetry of the arms. 2) The symmetry of the hands and the legs. 3) Whip like movements. 4) Physically balanced movements. 5) Condensing and extending movements. 6) Upper body symmetry. 7) Connected movements. 8) Shifting your weight gradually.

In the description of the movements, we will face South as the reference point for the starting position. Chart 3-1 is the movement chart with foot prints and directional arrows to assist your learning. On the chart there is a large area covered by movements, when in fact, the entire sequence is done overlapping in a long rectangular space. For the sake of clarity, we have drawn the movements above each other instead of overlapping.

We have intentionally taken the photographs from the rear view to ease your learning. In the placement of the photographs, we have also intentionally placed the sequence in the direction that you will be moving while learning the movements. Therefore, you will notice that sometimes the photographs are sequenced from left to right and sometimes from right to left. Bold arrows are placed next to the photos to indicate the overall direction of the movements. Where there is a reversal of direction, it will be indicated with a turning arrow where applicable.

Learn one posture at a time until it is smooth, then go on to the next posture. You may also wish to learn the hand and the leg movements separately to simplify your learning.

1. The symmetry of the arms: Pay attention to both hands when practicing Taijiquan. When one hand finishes a movement, the other hand finishes as well. This will allow an energetic symmetry to the arms (using physical symmetry to attain energetic symmetry).

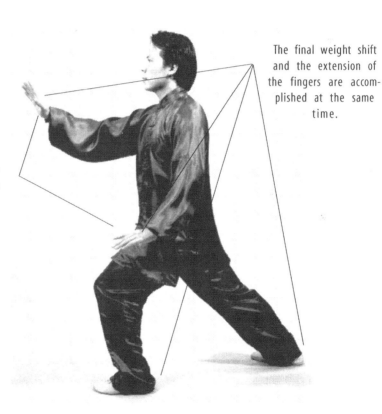

The final weight shift and the extension of the fingers are accomplished at the same time.

Hands settle into place at the same time

2. The symmetry of the hands and legs: When the legs complete a movement, the hands should also complete the movement at the same time. This will allow an energetic symmetry between the upper limbs and lower limbs.

41

3. Whip like movements (Stretch the arm): "Sink the shoulders, drop the elbows, settle the wrist, and extend the fingers". In this order, it trains you to lead the qi to your finger tips. It also allows the energy to flow smoothly from your torso to your finger tips.

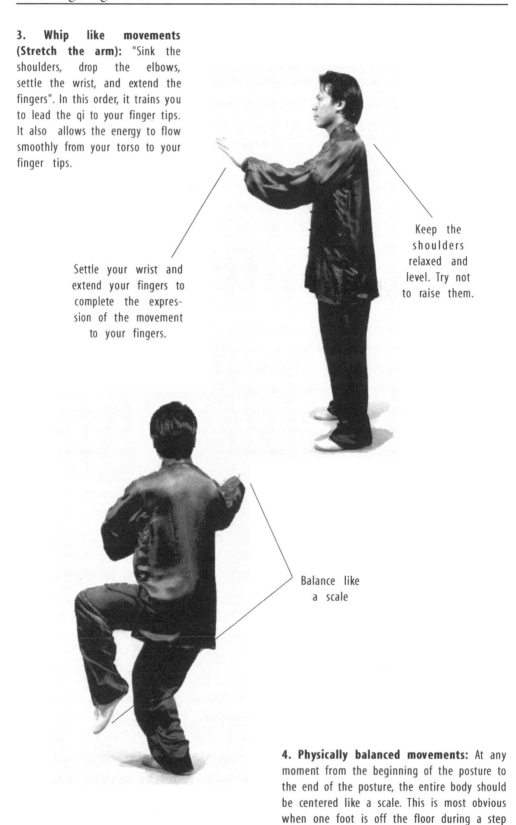

Keep the shoulders relaxed and level. Try not to raise them.

Settle your wrist and extend your fingers to complete the expression of the movement to your fingers.

Balance like a scale

4. Physically balanced movements: At any moment from the beginning of the posture to the end of the posture, the entire body should be centered like a scale. This is most obvious when one foot is off the floor during a step and while standing on one leg.

5. Condensing (yin) and extending (yang) movements (dynamic equilibrium, or pumping action): The different parts of the body should be in constant motion. In the Taijiquan routine, the entire body is constantly in motion. When any part of the body remains in a static condition for an extended time, then there is no yin-yang dynamic balancing action .

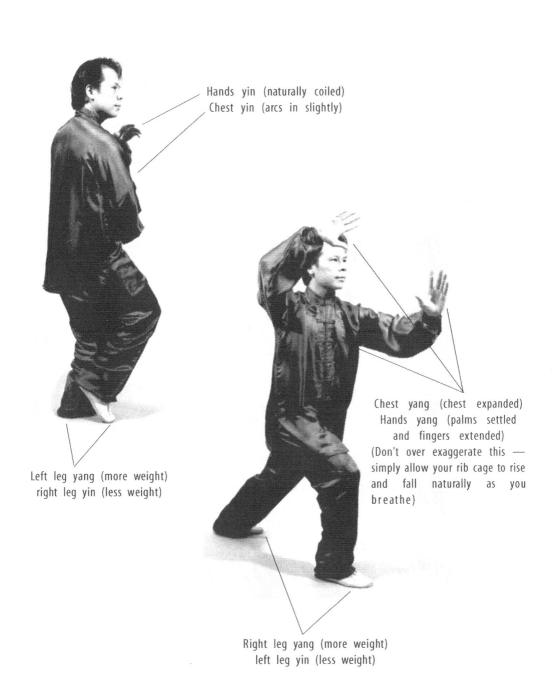

Hands yin (naturally coiled)
Chest yin (arcs in slightly)

Chest yang (chest expanded)
Hands yang (palms settled
and fingers extended)
(Don't over exaggerate this —
simply allow your rib cage to rise
and fall naturally as you
breathe)

Left leg yang (more weight)
right leg yin (less weight)

Right leg yang (more weight)
left leg yin (less weight)

6. Upper body symmetry: Keep the head straight, tongue touches the palate of your mouth, and breathe with the assistance of your abdomen. The top of your head (baihui) is a yang energy junction in your body. The bottom of the torso (huiyin) is a yin energy junction in your body. By keeping your head straight and paying attention to your abdominal area (breathing with your abdomen), this allows the torso to have a vertical balanced energy symmetry.

In Taijiquan practice, initially the breathing should be natural, following the pattern you are accustomed to. Don't pay too much attention to abdominal breathing until your overall movement has become smooth.

Keep head and body upright

Breathe with the assistance of your abdomen

Movement expressed through the fingers

7. Connected movements (Stretch the entire body): "Root at the feet, movement initiated by the legs, directed by the waist, and expressed through the fingers."

Movement initiated by the legs

Movement directed by the waist

Root at the feet

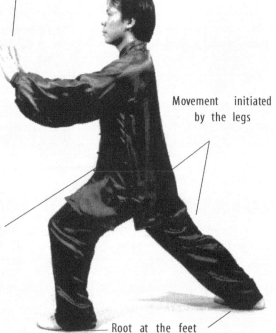

8. Shift your weight gradually: All movements are well balanced and controlled. When practicing this routine, shift your weight from one leg to the next without any abrupt changes in your movement. That is, don't fall into your stance.

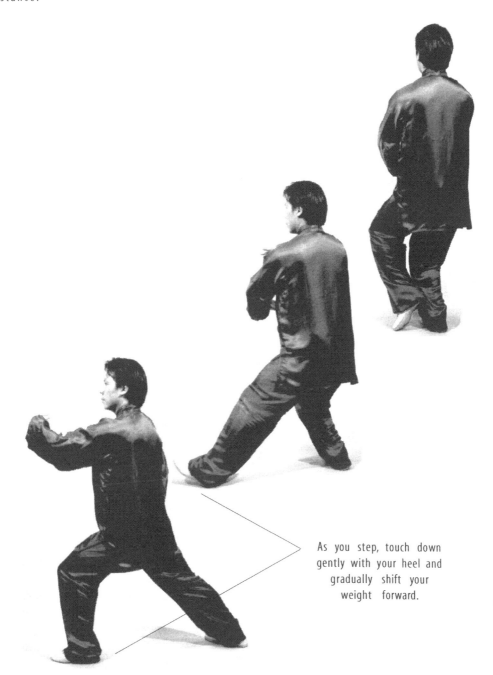

As you step, touch down gently with your heel and gradually shift your weight forward.

45

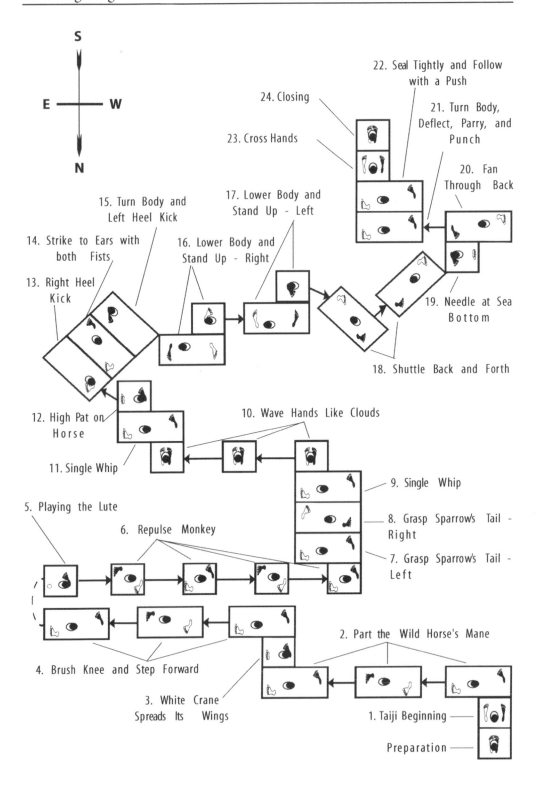

S

E — W

N

22. Seal Tightly and Follow with a Push

24. Closing

21. Turn Body, Deflect, Parry, and Punch

23. Cross Hands

20. Fan Through Back

15. Turn Body and Left Heel Kick

17. Lower Body and Stand Up - Left

14. Strike to Ears with both Fists

16. Lower Body and Stand Up - Right

13. Right Heel Kick

19. Needle at Sea Bottom

18. Shuttle Back and Forth

12. High Pat on Horse

10. Wave Hands Like Clouds

11. Single Whip

9. Single Whip

5. Playing the Lute

8. Grasp Sparrow's Tail - Right

6. Repulse Monkey

7. Grasp Sparrow's Tail - Left

2. Part the Wild Horse's Mane

4. Brush Knee and Step Forward

3. White Crane Spreads Its Wings

1. Taiji Beginning

Preparation

Chart 3-1: 24 Posture Taijiquan Movement Chart

24 Posture Tai Chi Chuan — List of Postures

1. Taiji Beginning 起勢
2. Part the Wild Horse's Mane 左右野馬分鬃
3. White Crane Spreads Its Wings 白鶴亮翅
4. Brush Knee and Step Forward 左右摟膝拗步
5. Playing the Lute 手揮琵琶
6. Repulse Monkey 左右倒攆猴
7. Grasp Sparrow's Tail - Left 左攬雀尾
8. Grasp Sparrow's Tail - Right 右攬雀尾
9. Single Whip 單鞭
10. Wave Hands Like Clouds 雲手
11. Single Whip 單鞭
12. High Pat on Horse 高探馬
13. Right Heel Kick 右蹬腳
14. Strike to Ears with Both Fists 雙峰貫耳
15. Turn Body and Left Heel Kick 轉身左蹬腳
16. Lower Body and Stand on One Leg - Left 左下勢獨立
17. Lower Body and Stand on One Leg - Right 右下勢獨立
18. Shuttle Back and Forth 左右穿梭
19. Needle at Sea Bottom 海底針
20. Fan Through Back 閃通背
21. Turn Body, Deflect, Parry, and Punch 轉身搬攔捶
22. Seal Tightly and Follow with a Push 如封似閉
23. Cross Hands 十字手
24. Closing 收勢

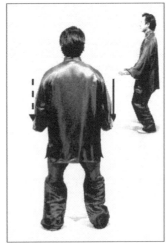 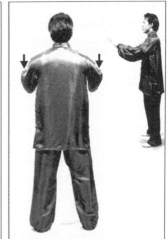

Figure 3-5   Figure 3-4

3.2. Twenty-Four Posture Taijiquan

Preparation

Movements:

Step 1. Stand with your feet together and your hands at your sides. (Figure 3-1, Face South)

Step 2. Mentally relax the front of your body from your head down to your toes. Relax one section at a time as you exhale to the section of intent.

Follow the same procedure and relax the back of your body. Finally, take a deep breath, exhale and relax from your head all the way down to your toes.

Notes:

1. Training the mind is of the highest importance in Taijiquan. The Preparation posture is for preparing the mind for the physical movements.

2. Before starting the movements, the mind should be in a calm abiding state. Stand naturally upright, bring your thoughts inward with your eyes looking evenly forward.

3. Since the breathing process is accomplished by contracting the intercostal muscles and the diaphragm, it is easier to exhale

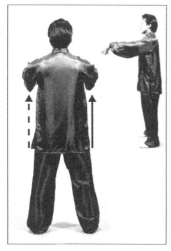
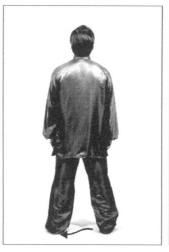
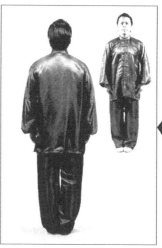

S
T
A
R
T

H
E
R
E

Figure 3-3   Figure 3-2   Figure 3-1

to relax the body than to inhale. Also, the intention is inward during an inhalation, where as the intention is on expansion during an exhalation, which also makes it easier for the body to relax.

Posture 1: Taiji Beginning

Movements: (Figures 3-2 to 3-5)

Step 1. Gently touch your tongue to the roof of your mouth.

Step 2. Bend your knees slightly, then step to your left with your left leg, shoulder width apart (Figure 3-2). Rotate your hands so your palms face down as you raise your arms up slowly to shoulder level (Figure 3-3).

Step 3. Pull your arms in slightly by bending your elbows, and lower your hands to your abdomen level, while you bend your knees and lower your body (Figures 3-4 and 3-5).

Notes:

1. When moving your arms up, don't raise your shoulders. Right before your hands reach shoulder level, bend your knees and begin lowering your elbows, while allowing your hands to continue to raise up to shoulder level. This will prevent the lifting of your shoulders and create a wave like movement in your arms, making the movements rounded and smooth.

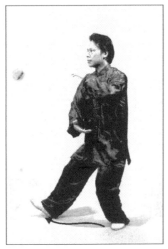 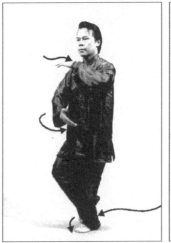 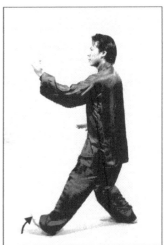

Figure 3-11　　　　　　Figure 3-10　　　　　　Figure 3-9

2. The bending of your knees and the lowering of your hands should be done simultaneously. Do not bend your knees excessively. Go as low as you can, without leaning forward. Your weight should be evenly distributed between your legs.

4. When raising your arms, your hands should be in a naturally relaxed position. When lowering your arms, gently settle your palms and extend your fingers as you complete the posture. This shows a continuation and expression of movement to your fingers.

Posture 2: Part the Wild Horse's Mane

Movements: (Figures 3-6 to 3-16)

Step 1. *Left*: Gradually shift your weight to your right foot while turning your body slightly to your right, then back to face forward. At the same time, bring your left foot next to your right foot, while circling both hands counterclockwise and rotating them to face each other (Figure 3-6).

The hands and arms resemble the embracing of a ball (Taiji Ball) in front of your chest.

Step 2. Step to your left with your left foot, touching down with your heel first. (Figure 3-7, Step East).

Turn towards your left, while pulling your right hand down and extending your left hand forward as you shift

50

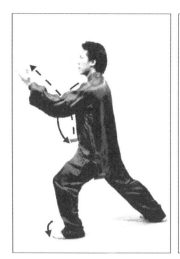

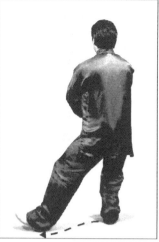

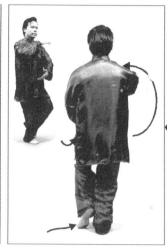

Figure 3-8   Figure 3-7   Figure 3-6

your weight forward into a left Bow Stance (Figure 3-8, Face East).

At the completion of this posture, your left palm faces up at an angle between your shoulder and eye level, and your right palm faces down at your hip level.

Step 3. *Right*: Shift your weight back to your right foot and lift the ball of your left foot up (Figure 3-9).

Turn your body and left foot outwards and shift all your weight on to your left foot and bring your right foot next to your left foot. At the same time, rotate your hands until your palms are facing each other in the Hold the Taiji Ball position. (Figure 3-10).

Step 4. Step forward with your right foot, touching down with your heel first (Figure 3-11).

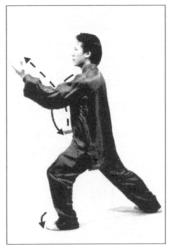 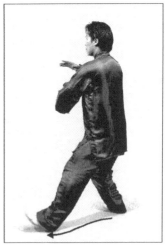

Figure 3-16   Figure 3-15

Shift your weight forward into a right Bow Stance, while extending your right hand, palm forward and up, and lowering your left hand, palm facing down until it is next to your hip (Figure 3-12, Face East)

Step 5. *Left*: Shift your weight back to your left foot. Lift the ball of your right foot up (Figure 3-13).

Turn your body and right foot outwards and shift all your weight on to your right foot and bring your left foot next to your right foot. At the same time, rotate your hands until your palms are facing each other in the Hold the Taiji Ball position. (Figure 3-14).

Step 6. Repeat Step 2. Step to your left with your left foot, touching down with your heel first. (Figure 3-15, Step East).

Turn towards your left, while pulling your right hand down and extending your left hand forward as you shift your weight forward into a left Bow Stance (Figure 3-16, Face East).

At the completion of this posture, your left palm faces up at an angle between your shoulder and eye level, and your right palm faces down at your hip level.

Notes:

1. When holding the Taiji Ball in front of your chest, keep your right elbow lower than your shoulder, to prevent unnecessary

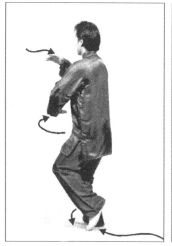 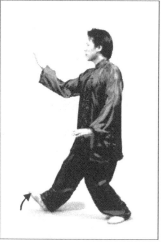 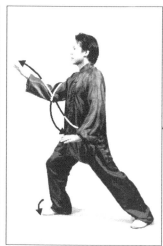

S
T
A
R
T

H
E
R
E

Figure 3-14   Figure 3-13   Figure 3-12

tension on your shoulder. The hands are in a naturally relaxed position.

When holding the Taiji Ball, "Arc the chest and round the back" slightly. Release the arc when you extend your arms. This is a condensing and extending action of the chest and back, which also provides a gentle massage to the internal organs.

While learning this routine, in the beginning, don't be too concerned with this. Simply giving some awareness to the elastic like movements of the rib cage will suffice.

2. When stepping to your left with your left foot, from the holding the Taiji Ball position, don't turn your body too early. Turning your body before your left foot is planted, may create unnecessary torsion on the right knee. The turning should be accomplished with the waist and hips, not the knees.

On the other hand, don't turn your body too late. Turning your body after you have completed the shifting of your weight forward, will create a discontinuity of motion.

3. The length of your step is restricted by how low your weighted foot is able to bend. It is not necessary to take a very long step. A long step will have the tendency to tense the rest of your body unnecessarily, and may cause your body to lean.

4. At the completion of this posture, the leg position is referred to as Bow Stance. The weight distribution is about 70% on the front leg and 30% on the back leg.

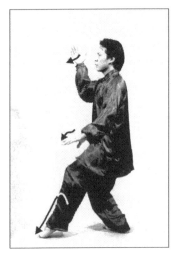
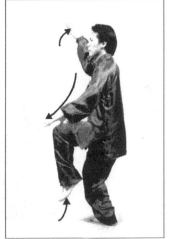

| Figure 3-21 | Figure 3-20 |

If we were to draw a line from the front to the back, your front foot and back foot should be on either side of the line. This will provide better balance than if both feet were on the line. To accomplish this, when you step, step slightly off to the side.

Also, the angle formed with the front foot and back foot should not exceed 90 degrees. When necessary, turn your back foot in. While in the Bow Stance, your front knee should not go past your toes in order to prevent undue stress on your knee.

5. When stepping into Bow Stance, the heel touches down first, then gradually turn your body as you shift about 70% of your weight to the front leg. Do not fall into the stance. That is, there should be no abrupt changes in movement. As the back leg extends until it is straight, but not locked, the hands should also complete their extension.

6. At the completion of this posture, settle your lower wrist slightly and extend the fingers, and extend the fingers of your front hand slightly.

Posture 3: White Crane Spreads Its Wings

Movements: (Figures 3-17 to 3-21)

Step 1. Shift all your weight onto your left foot while bringing your right foot behind your left (Figure 3-17). Shift your

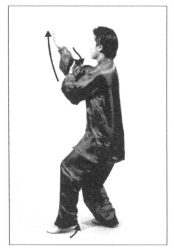
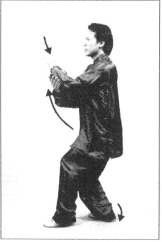
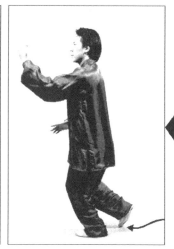

S
T
A
R
T

H
E
R
E

Figure 3-19   Figure 3-18   Figure 3-17

weight completely onto your right foot and turn your body slightly to your left while extending your right hand, palm up under your left forearm (Figure 3-18)

Step 2. Turn your body towards your right slightly as you raise your right arm up towards your right and lower your left hand, palm down, toward your right elbow (Figure 3-19).

Continue raising your right arm and lowering your left arm. At the same time, rotate your left palm to face down and raise your left foot completely off the floor (Figure 3-20).

Step 3. Turn your body to face forward. Touch down with the ball of your left foot into an Empty Stance and settle your wrists (Figure 3-21).

Notes:

1. From the Part the Wild Horse's Mane posture, the movement of the right hand draws a semicircular path from your bottom right to your upper right.

2. White Crane Spreads Its Wings describes the beauty of the crane's wings. When you wear the traditional Chinese white outfit to do this posture, it appears as though you are a crane spreading its wings. It is very pleasing to the eyes.

3. At the completion of this posture, both arms should have a rounded feeling to them.

55

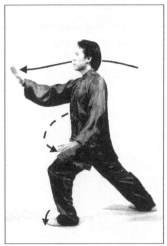 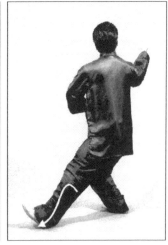

Figure 3-26   Figure 3-25

Posture 4: Brush Knee and Step Forward

Movements: (Figures 3-22 to 3-35)

Step 1. Turn your body towards your left while rotating your right hand so your palm faces you (Figure 3-22). Then turn your body towards your right, while lowering your right hand and circling your left hand up (Figure 3-23)

Continue to turn your body towards your right as you raise your right hand up and lower your left hand. At the same time, raise your left foot off the floor (Figure 3-24)

Step 2. *Left*: Step forward with your left foot, touching down with your heel first (Figure 3-25).

Brush your left hand across your left knee and extend your right hand forward as you shift your weight to your left foot into Bow Stance (Figure 3-26).

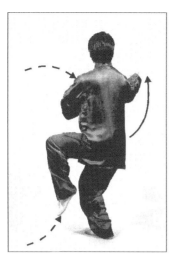

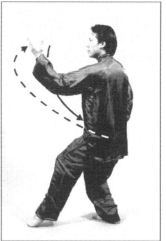

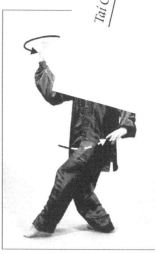

H
E
R
E

| Figure 3-24 | Figure 3-23 | Figure 3-22 |

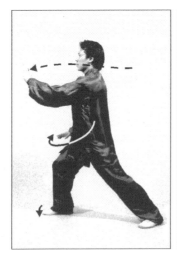 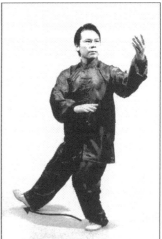

Figure 3-31   Figure 3-30

Step 3. *Right*: Shift your weight back to your right foot (Figure 3-27). Turn your body to your left and rotate your right hand, so your palm faces to your left, and lower your left hand (Figure 3-28).

Shift all your weight onto your left foot and bring your right foot forward next to your left. At the same time, begin to lower your right hand, palm down in front of your body and raise your left hand, palm up, to head level (Figure 3-29).

Step 4. Step forward with your right foot, touching down with your heel first, as you continue to lower your right hand, palm down, and raise your left hand (Figure 3-30).

Shift your weight to your right foot into Bow Stance as you brush your right palm across your right knee and extend your left hand forward (Figure 3-31).

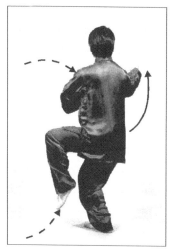

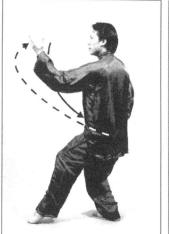

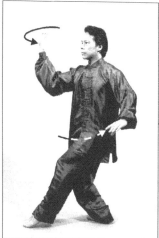

S
T
A
R
T

H
E
R
E

Figure 3-24

Figure 3-23

Figure 3-22

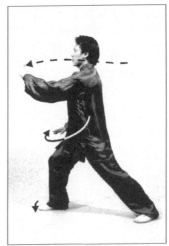 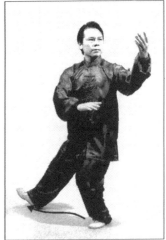

Figure 3-31   Figure 3-30

Step 3. *Right*: Shift your weight back to your right foot (Figure 3-27). Turn your body to your left and rotate your right hand, so your palm faces to your left, and lower your left hand (Figure 3-28).

Shift all your weight onto your left foot and bring your right foot forward next to your left. At the same time, begin to lower your right hand, palm down in front of your body and raise your left hand, palm up, to head level (Figure 3-29).

Step 4. Step forward with your right foot, touching down with your heel first, as you continue to lower your right hand, palm down, and raise your left hand (Figure 3-30).

Shift your weight to your right foot into Bow Stance as you brush your right palm across your right knee and extend your left hand forward (Figure 3-31).

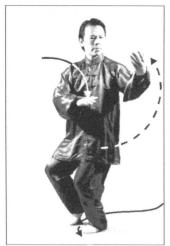

Figure 3-29

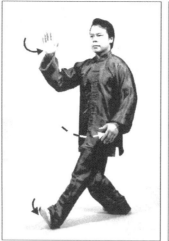

Figure 3-28

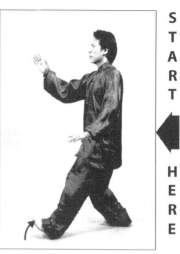

Figure 3-27

START HERE

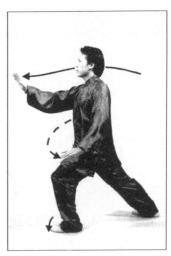

Figure 3-35

Step 5. *Left*: Shift your weight back to your left foot (Figure 3-32). Turn your right foot out about 45 degrees and shift all your weight on it; and bring your left foot forward next to your right foot. At the same time begin to lower your left hand, palm down, in front of your body and raise your right hand, palm up (Figure 3-33).

Step 6. Repeat Step 2. Step forward with your left foot, touching down with your heel first (Figure 3-34).

Brush your left hand across your left knee and extend your right hand forward as you shift your weight to your left foot into Bow Stance (Figure 3-35).

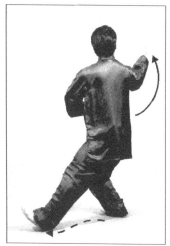 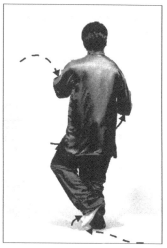 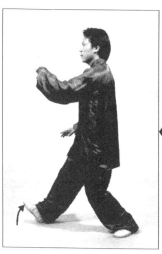

S
T
A
R
T

H
E
R
E

Figure 3-34   Figure 3-33   Figure 3-32

Note:

1. Don't shift your weight forward too quickly. Allow your upper hand to be in front of your body before you complete your final weight shift forward.

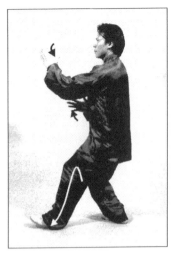

Figure 3-39

Posture 5: Playing the Lute

Movements: (Figures 3-36 to 3-39)

Step 1. Shift your weight forward and bring your right foot a half step forward (Figure 3-36). Shift all your weight back to your right foot and rotate both hands to face in (Figure 3-37).

Step 2. Lift your left foot up and touch down with your heel, while circling your right hand down and circling your left hand forward. Then gently press in with your palms towards the center and relax your arms out slightly (Figures 3-38 and 3-39).

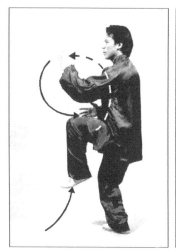
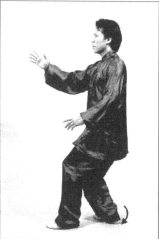
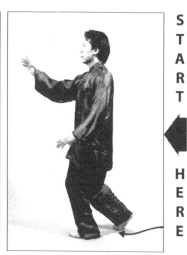

Figure 3-38   Figure 3-37   Figure 3-36

Note:

1. When making the half step with your right foot, touch down with the ball of your foot first, then gradually shift your weight on it.

S
T
A
R
T

➤

H
E
R
E

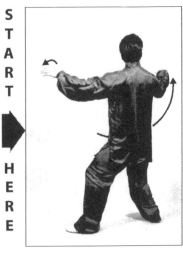

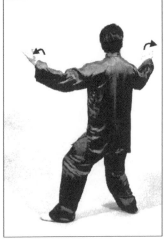

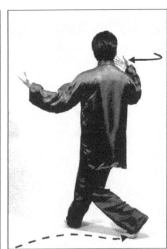

Figure 3-40   Figure 3-41   Figure 3-42

Posture 6: Repulse Monkey

Movements: (Figures 3-40 to 3-55)

Step 1. Put the ball of your left foot down and begin to lower your right arm.

Step 2. *Right*: Extend your right arm behind you and left arm forward with both palms facing down (Figure 3-40).

Turn your body towards your back hand as you drop both elbows and rotate both hands, so your palms face up (Figure 3-41).

Begin turning your body towards your left as you bend your right elbow and begin extending your right hand forward. At the same time, step back with your left foot (Figure 3-42).

Continue to turn your body towards your left as you extend your right hand forward and draw your left hand, palm up, down to your waist. At the same time, shift your weight back to your left foot, as you pivot on the ball of your right foot and turn your right heel towards your right (Figure 3-43).

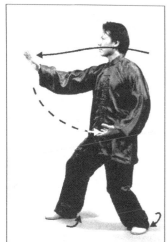
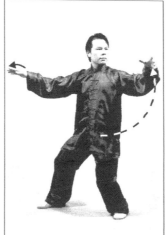
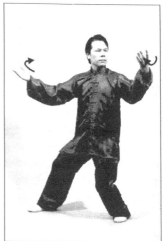

Figure 3-43   Figure 3-44   Figure 3-45

Step 3. *Left*: Extend your left arm behind you and right arm
forward with both palms facing down (Figure 3-44).

Turn your body towards your back hand as you drop
both elbows and rotate both hands so your palms face up
(Figure 3-45).

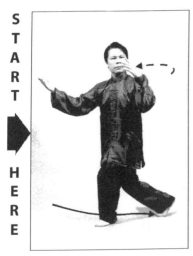

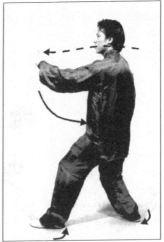

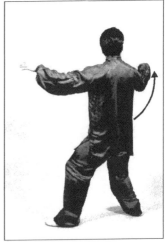

Figure 3-46	Figure 3-47	Figure 3-48

Begin turning your body towards your right as you bend your left elbow and begin extending your left hand forward. At the same time, step back with your right foot (Figure 3-46).

Continue to turn your body towards your right as you extend your left hand forward and draw your right hand, palm up, down to your waist. At the same time, shift your weight back to your right foot, pivot on the ball of your left foot and turn your left heel towards your left (Figure 3-47).

Step 4. *Right*: Repeat Step 2. Extend your right arm behind you and left arm forward with both palms facing down (Figure 3-48).

Turn your body towards your back hand as you drop both elbows and rotate both hands, so your palms face up (Figure 3-49).

Begin turning your body towards your left as you bend your right elbow and begin extending your right hand forward. At the same time, step back with your left foot (Figure 3-50).

Continue to turn your body towards your left as you extend your right hand forward and draw your left hand, palm up, down to your waist. At the same time, shift your weight back to your left foot, as you pivot on the ball of your right foot and turn your right heel towards your right (Figure 3-51).

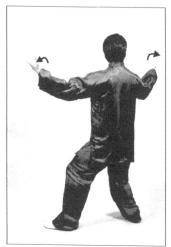

Figure 3-49

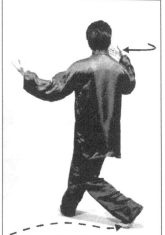

Figure 3-50

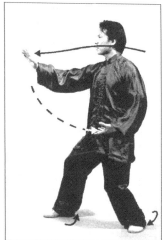

Figure 3-51

S
T
A
R
T

H
E
R
E

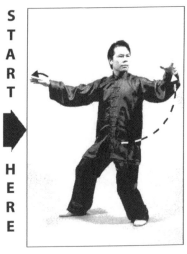

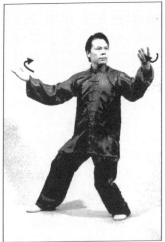

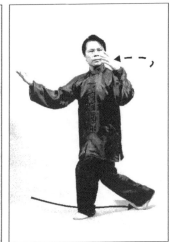

Figure 3-52

Figure 3-53

Figure 3-54

Step 5. *Left*: Repeat Step 3. Extend your left arm behind you and right arm forward with both palms facing down (Figure 3-52).

Turn your body towards your back hand as you drop both elbows and rotate both hands so your palms face up (Figure 3-53).

Begin turning your body towards your right as you bend your left elbow and begin extending your left hand forward. At the same time, step back with your right foot (Figure 3-54).

Continue to turn your body towards your right as you extend your left hand forward and draw your right hand, palm up, down to your waist. At the same time, shift your weight back to your right foot, pivot on the ball of your left foot and turn your left heel towards your left (Figure 3-55).

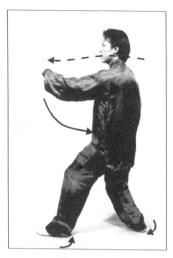

Figure 3-55

Notes:

1. Extend your arms back only as far as the turning of your hips and waist permit. Do not turn from your knees.

2. When stepping back, touch down on the ball of your foot first, then gradually shift your weight on it. At the same time, pivot with the ball of your front foot as you turn your body.

3. Don't cross your legs when you step backward. Remember to keep your feet on either side of an imaginary line.

4. Your eyes should follow the movement of the more active hand (the hand that is extending forward).

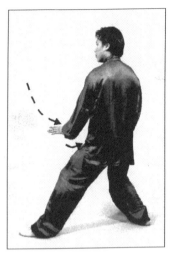
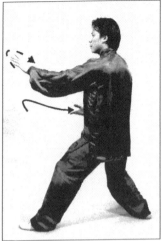
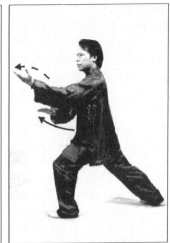

Figure 3-61   Figure 3-60   Figure 3-59

Posture 7: Grasp the Sparrow's Tail - Left

Movements: (Figures 3-56 to 3-68)

Step 1. Shift all your weight back to your right foot and bring your feet together. At the same time, circle your right hand up and in as you lower your left hand down and in. Your hands should finish in the holding the Taiji Ball position with your palms facing each other (Figure 3-56).

Step 2. *Ward Off*: Step forward with your left foot, touching down with your heel first (Figure 57, Step East).

Turn your body forward as you shift your weight forward into a left Bow Stance. At the same time, pull your right hand down and extend your left forearm forward and up (Figure 3-58).

Step 3. *Roll Back*: Turn your body slightly towards your left as you extend both hands towards your front left corner. At the same time, rotate your left hand so your palm faces up (Figure 3-59).

Shift your weight back. At the same time, rotate both hands clockwise by making small circles with your hands and begin pulling your arms back towards your body (Figures 3-60 and 3-61).

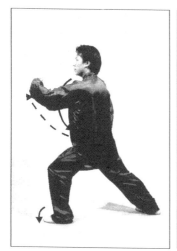

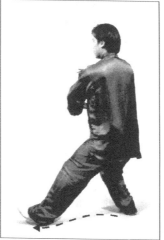

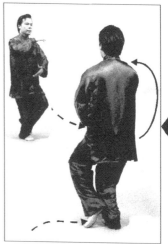

S
T
A
R
T

H
E
R
E

Figure 3-58   Figure 3-57   Figure 3-56

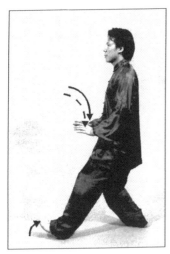
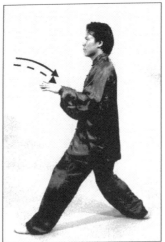
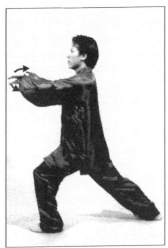

Figure 3-67   Figure 3-66   Figure 3-65

Step 4. *Press*: Lower both hands down and up to the back (Figure 3-62). Turn your body to face forward as you bring your right hand, palm facing out, next to your left hand, palm facing in (Figure 3-63).

Touch your right palm to your left wrist, and press both palms forward, while shifting your weight to your left foot (Figure 3-64). Left palm faces in and right palm faces out.

Step 5. *Push*: Rotate both hands so your palms face down (Figure 3-65). Shift your weight to your back foot as you separate your hands and begin pulling them back towards your body (Figure 3-66).

Shift your weight back further and lift the ball of your front foot up while pushing down with both hands toward your abdomen (Figure 3-67).

Push forward with both hands while shifting your weight to your left foot (Figure 3-68). The hands draw a small pear shape as you push forward.

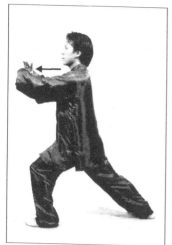

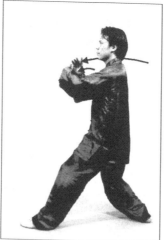

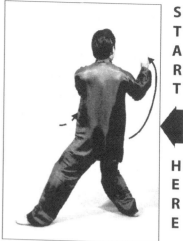

S
T
A
R
T

H
E
R
E

Figure 3-64   Figure 3-63   Figure 3-62

Note:

1. Pay attention to how you shift your weight and turn your waist. Allow the arms to move wherever the waist directs them to go. Don't overextend your arms by locking your shoulders or turn your upper body by torquing your knees.

S
T
A
R
T

➤

H
E
R
E

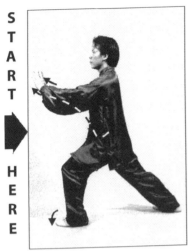

Figure 3-68

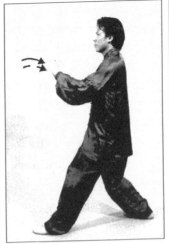

Figure 3-69

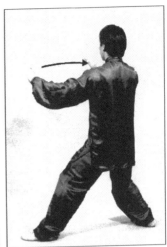

Figure 3-70

Posture 8: Grasp the Sparrow's Tail - Right

Movements: (Figures 3-69 to 3-84)

Step 1. Shift your weight back to your right foot (Figure 3-69). Turn your body to your right as you turn your left foot in and right foot out. At the same time, extend your right arm to your right, and lower your left arm slightly (Figures 3-70 and 3-71).

Shift all your weight back to your left foot and bring your right foot next to your left foot. At the same time, lower your right hand down to abdomen level and bring your left hand in front of your chest. You should now be in a holding the Taiji Ball position (Figure 3-72).

Step 2. *Ward Off*: Step forward with your right foot, touching down with your heel first (Figure 73, Step West).

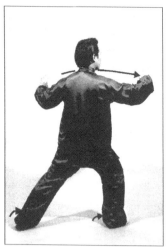
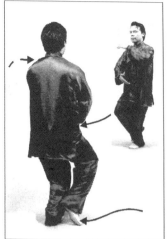
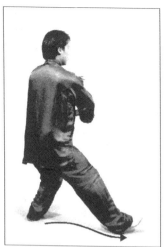

Figure 3-71   Figure 3-72   Figure 3-73

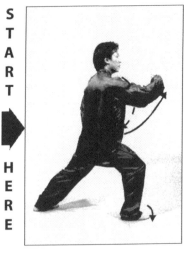
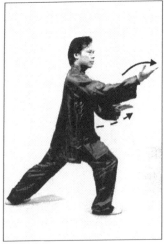
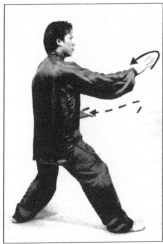

S
T
A
R
T

➤

H
E
R
E

Figure 3-74   Figure 3-75   Figure 3-76

Turn your body forward as you shift your weight forward into a right Bow Stance. At the same time, pull your right hand down and extend your left forearm forward and up (Figure 3-74).

Step 3. *Roll Back*: Turn your body slightly towards your right as you extend both hands towards your front right corner. At the same time, rotate your right hand so your palm faces up (Figure 3-75).

Shift your weight back. At the same time rotate both hands counterclockwise by making small circles with your hands and begin pulling your arms back towards your body (Figures 3-76 and 3-77).

Step 4. *Press*: Lower both hands down and up to the back (Figure 3-78). Turn your body to face forward as you bring your left palm next to your right wrist (Figure 3-79).

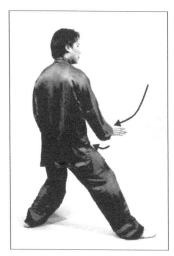

Figure 3-77

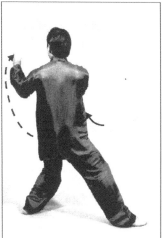

Figure 3-78

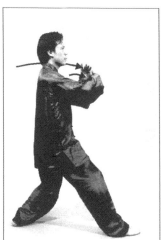

Figure 3-79

S
T
A
R
T

H
E
R
E

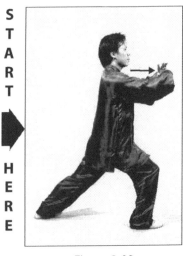

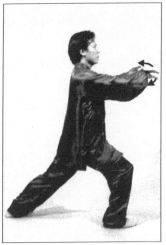

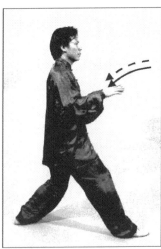

Figure 3-80   Figure 3-81   Figure 3-82

Touch your left palm to your right wrist, and press both palms forward, while shifting your weight to your right foot (Figure 3-80). Right palm faces in and left palm face out.

Step 5. *Push*: Rotate both hands so your palms face down (Figure 3-81). Shift your weight to your back foot as you separate your hands and begin pulling them towards your body (Figure 3-82).

Shift your weight back further and lift the ball of your front foot up while pushing down with both hands toward your abdomen (Figure 3-83).

Push forward with both hands while shifting your weight to your right foot (Figure 3-84). The hands draw a small pear shape as you push forward.

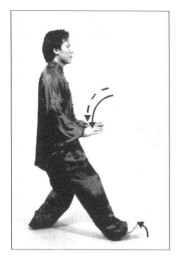
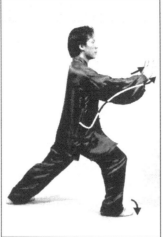

Figure 3-83   Figure 3-84

Notes:

1. Same notes as in Posture 7.

2. Whenever you turn your body around 180 degrees, allow your back foot to pivot out as necessary, to prevent undue torsion on your knee. As your hips and waist become more flexible, it may no longer be necessary to turn your foot out.

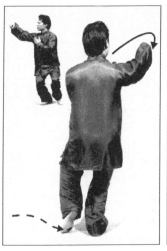
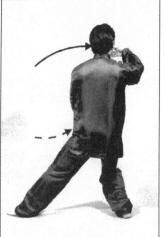
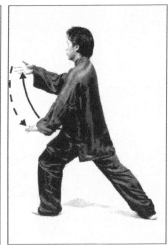

Figure 3-90   Figure 3-89   Figure 3-88

Posture 9: Single Whip

Movements: (Figures 3-85 to 3-97)

Step 1. Shift your weight back to your left foot and turn your right foot in. At the same time, begin turning your body towards your left while rotating both hands so your palms face out (Figures 3-85 and 3-86).

Continue to turn your body towards your left and bring your left arm across your body to your left, then down, while lowering your right arm down then up (Figures 3-87 and 3-88).

Step 2. Shift your weight back completely to your right foot and bring your left foot next to your right foot. At the same time, turn to your right and hook down with your right hand while bringing your left hand next to your right shoulder (Figures 3-89 and 3-90).

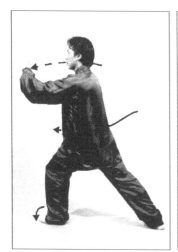

Figure 3-87

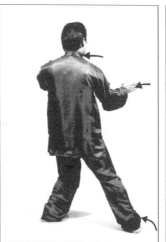

Figure 3-86

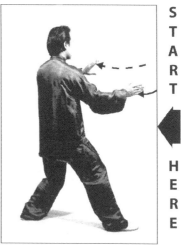

Figure 3-85

S
T
A
R
T

HERE

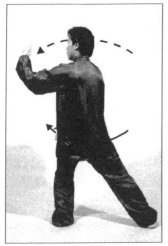
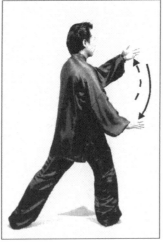
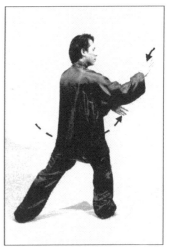

Figure 3-96   Figure 3-95   Figure 3-94

Step to your left with your left foot, and begin to rotate and extend your left hand forward (Figure 3-91). Shift your weight to your left foot and complete your left palm rotation outward and extend your hand forward (Figure 3-92, Face East).

Notes:

1. Single Whip is referring to the motion of a whip, with the body of the whip moving forward and backward before snapping forward.

2. When you complete this posture, keep your right elbow slightly bent, align your left elbow with your left knee, and keep both shoulders relaxed.

3. When rotating and extending your left hand, it should be completed with the turning of your body.

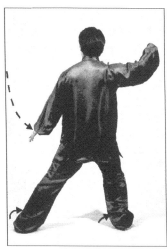 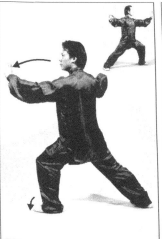 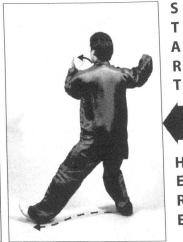

Figure 3-93   Figure 3-92   Figure 3-91

Posture 10: Wave Hands Like Clouds

Movements: (Figures 3-93 to 3-110)

Step 1. Shift your weight back to your right foot as you turn your left foot in and right foot out. At the same time, lower your left hand down and up towards the right side of your chest, and open your right hand and begin lowering it (Figures 3-93 and 3-94)

Step 2. Move your right hand down to your hip level and your left hand up to your eye level (Figure 3-95). Turn your body towards your left and shift your weight to your left foot (Figure 3-96).

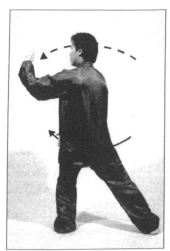 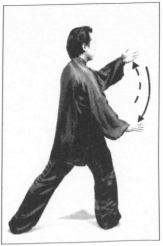 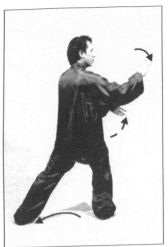

Figure 3-102   Figure 3-101   Figure 3-100

Bring your right foot close to your left foot while settling your left wrist and beginning to bring your right arm up towards your chest (Figure 3-97).

Step 3. Move your left hand down to your hip level and your right hand up to your eye level (Figure 3-98). Turn your body towards your right and shift your weight to your right foot (Figure 3-99).

Step to your left with your left foot, while settling your right wrist, and beginning to bring your left arm up towards your chest (Figure 3-100).

Step 4. Repeat Step 2. Move your right hand down to your hip level and your left hand up to your eye level (Figure 3-101). Turn your body towards your left and shift your weight to your left foot (Figure 3-102).

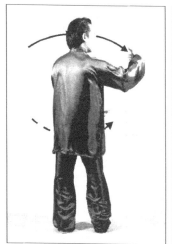

Figure 3-99

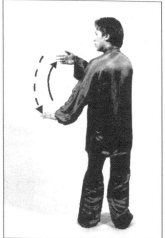

Figure 3-98

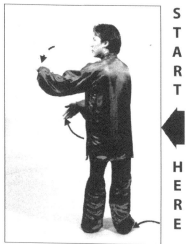

Figure 3-97

S
T
A
R
T

H
E
R
E

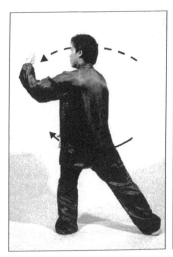

Figure 3-108

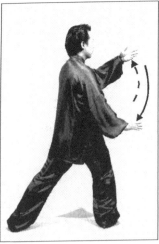

Figure 3-107

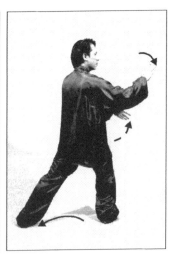

Figure 3-106

Bring your right foot close to your left foot while settling your left wrist and beginning to bring your right arm up towards your chest (Figure 3-103).

Step 5. Repeat Step 3. Move your left hand down to your hip level and your right hand up to your eye level (Figure 3-104). Turn your body towards your right and shift your weight to your right foot (Figure 3-105).

Step to your left with your left foot, while settling your right wrist, and beginning to bring your left arm up towards your chest (Figure 3-106).

Step 6. Repeat Step 2. Move your right hand down to your hip level and your left hand up to your eye level (Figure 3-107). Turn your body towards your left and shift your weight to your left foot (Figure 3-108).

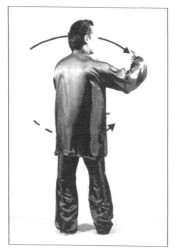

Figure 3-105

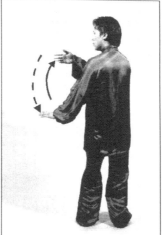

Figure 3-104

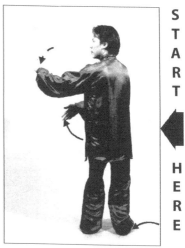

Figure 3-103

S
T
A
R
T

H
E
R
E

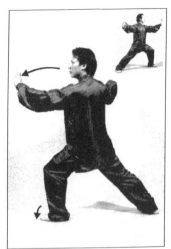 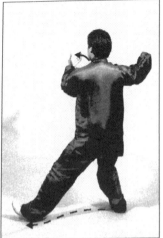 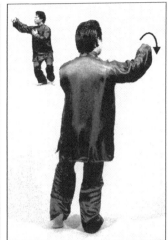

Figure 3-114   Figure 3-113   Figure 3-112

Bring your right foot close to your left foot while settling your left wrist and beginning to bring your right arm up towards your chest (Figure 3-109).

Step 7. Move your left hand down to your hip level and your right hand up to your eye level (Figure 3-110).

Notes:

1. Wave Hands Like Clouds is referring to the movement of the arms, as though they were clouds moving past each other — not touching and moving in unison.

2. Use your waist to direct the movement of your upper body.

3. Maintain one height as you step. Your arms should follow the movement of your waist.

4. Each hand draws a circle which overlaps in front of your body.

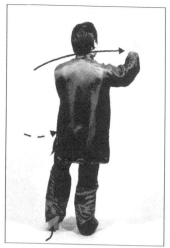
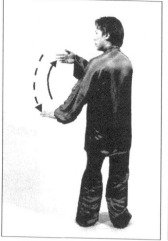
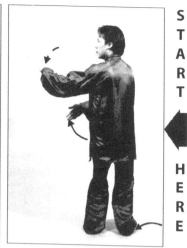

START HERE

Figure 3-111   Figure 3-110   Figure 3-109

Posture 11: Single Whip

Movements: (Figures 3-111 to 3-114)

Step 1. Turn your body towards your right and shift your weight to your right foot (Figure 3-111). Hook your right hand down and bring your left hand next to your right shoulder (Figure 3-112).

Step 2. Step to your left with your left foot, and begin to rotate and extend your left hand forward (Figure 3-113). Shift your weight to your left foot and complete your left palm rotation outward and extend your hand forward (Figure 3-114, Face East).

Note:

1. Same notes as in Posture 9.

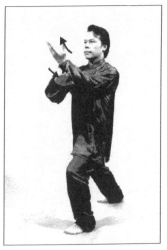
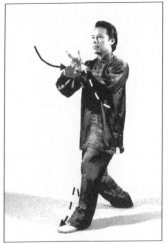
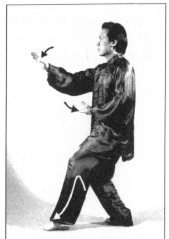

Figure 3-120	Figure 3-119	Figure 3-118

Posture 12: High Pat on Horse

Movements: (Figures 3-115 to 3-118)

Step 1. Shift your weight forward and bring your back foot forward behind your front foot. At the same time, rotate both hands so your palms face up (Figure 3-115)

Step 2. Shift all your weight back to your right foot. At the same time, begin to bring your front hand back and extend your back hand forward (Figure 3-116).

Bend your right elbow and extend your right hand forward, while pulling your left hand back towards your body with your palms facing each other. At the same time raise your left foot up than down. (Figures 3-117 and 3-118).

Notes:

1. High Pat on Horse is referring to a rider gauging the height of the horse's back before mounting.

2. Keep your body naturally erect and your shoulders relaxed.

3. When making the half step, maintain one height.

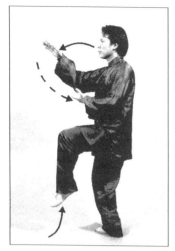
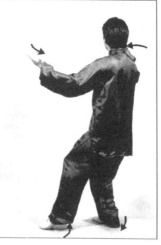
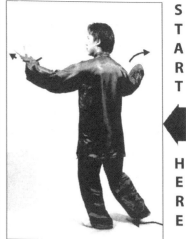

Figure 3-117   Figure 3-116   Figure 3-115

Posture 13: Right Heel Kick

Movements: (Figures 3-119 to 3-124)

Step 1. Turn slightly to face Northeast and take a small step in that direction (Figure 3-119) Shift your weight forward into a left Bow Stance as you extend your left hand over the back of your right hand (Figure 3-120).

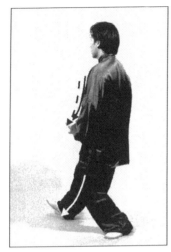
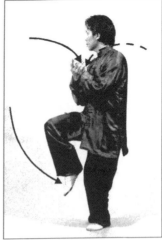
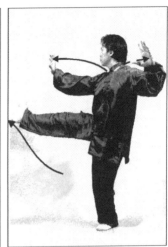

Figure 3-126   Figure 3-125   Figure 3-124

Continue to shift your weight from your right foot to your left and bring your right foot next to your left foot. At the same time, rotate your left hand so your palm faces down, circle both hands down then up, and cross them in front of your chest with your palms facing in (Figures 3-121 and 3-122).

Step 2. Lift your right foot up, and straighten your left leg (not locked) and extend your arms out to your sides with your palms facing out. At the same time, kick with your right heel to the Southeast direction (Figures 3-123 and 3-124).

Notes:

1. Extend your right hand in the same direction as your kick.

2. Kick only as high as you can without leaning your body.

3. When kicking with your right heel, don't lock your left knee.

4. The arm extension and the kick should be executed together. Your right arm and right leg should be aligned in the same vertical plane.

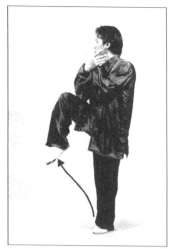

Figure 3-123

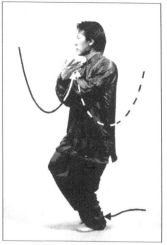

Figure 3-122

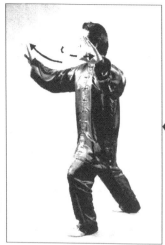

Figure 3-121

S
T
A
R
T

H
E
R
E

Posture 14: Strike to Ears With Both Fists

Movements: (Figures 3-125 to 3-127)

Step 1. Pull your right leg back and bring your forearms back and cross them in front of your chest, palms face in (Figure 3-125).

Lower your body by bending your left knee. At the same time turn to face Southeast and step down, while lowering your hands, palms face up, next to your abdomen (Figure 3-126).

S
T
A
R
T

→

H
E
R
E

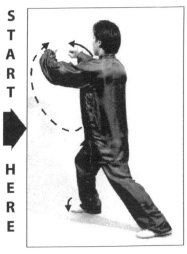

Figure 3-127

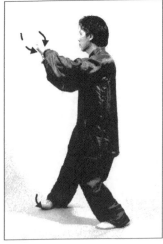

Figure 3-128

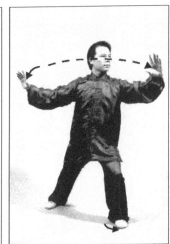

Figure 3-129

Step 2. Shift your weight forward into a right Bow Stance. At the same time, circle your hands to your sides then up as you change your hands into fists. The palms of your fists face forward (Figure 3-127).

Notes:

1. When stepping down with your right foot, bend your left knee slightly and place your right foot down gently.

2. Be careful to not extend your right knee past your right foot and don't lean forward.

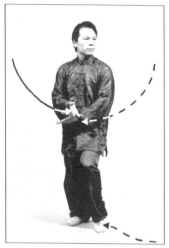

Figure 3-130

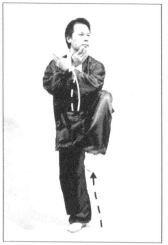

Figure 3-131

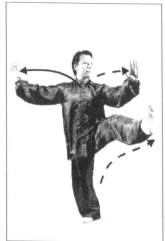

Figure 3-132

Posture 15: Turn Body and Left Heel Kick

Movements: (Figures 3-128 to 3-132)

Step 1. Shift your weight back, turn your right foot in and left foot out, as you turn your body 180 degree around. At the same time, open your fists and separate your arms to your sides (Figures 3-128 and 3-129).

Shift all your weight back to your right foot and bring your left foot back next to your right. At the same time, circle both hands down then up, until your forearms are crossed in front of your chest with your palms facing you. Left hand on the outside (Figure 3-130).

Step 2. Lift your left foot up, extend your arms to your sides with your palms facing out. At the same time, kick with your left heel in the Northwest direction (Figures 3-131 and 3-132).

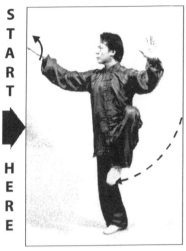 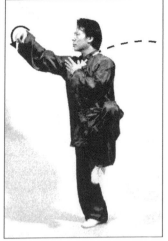 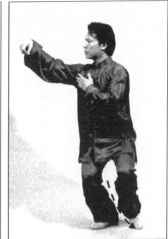

Figure 3-133   Figure 3-134   Figure 3-135

Posture 16: Lower Body Then Stand on One Leg - Left

Movements: (Figures 3-133 to 3-139)

Step 1. Pull your left foot back. Rotate your right palm to face up then down as you change your right hand into a hook. At the same time, bring your left hand back next to your right shoulder with your palm facing your chest (Figures 3-133 and 3-134).

   Begin lowering your body by bending your right knee (Figure 3-135).

Step 2. Step West with your left foot, as you lower your left hand towards your left foot (Figure 3-136).

Step 3. Shift your weight forward into a left Bow Stance, as you turn your front foot forward and back foot in. At the same time, extend your left hand forward then up in front of you, and lower your right hand down and rotate the hook to point up (Figure 3-137).

Step 4. Turn your left foot out slightly as you rotate your left hand so your palm faces down (Figure 3-138).

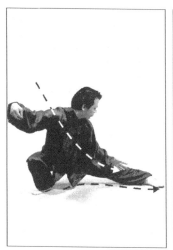

Figure 3-136

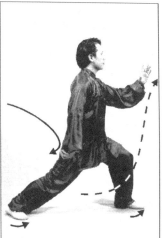

Figure 3-137

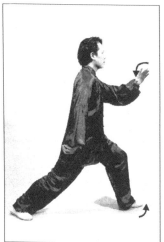

Figure 3-138

S
T
A
R
T

➤

H
E
R
E

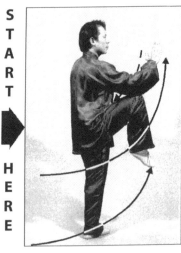

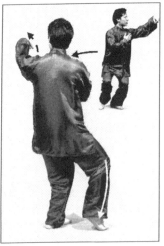

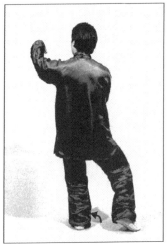

Figure 3-139   Figure 3-140   Figure 3-141

Shift all your weight forward onto your left foot and stand up, with your right knee as high as you can. At the same time, brush your left hand down to the side of your hip, with your palm facing down, and open your right hand and lift it up to eye level in front of you, with your palm facing to the left (Figure 3-139).

Notes:

1. This posture is made up of two parts: Snake Creeps Down and Golden Rooster Stands on One Leg.

2. When lowering your body, go only as low as you can without straining your bent knee. Also, keep your upper body as upright as you can.

3. As you lower your body, make sure that you bend your knee in the same direction as your foot.

3. When you stand up, the supporting leg shouldn't be locked.

4. When moving your leg up, imagine that your arm is controlling the lifting of your leg, as though there were a string attached to your leg and arm like a puppet.

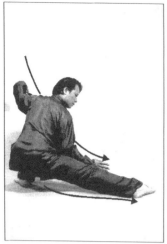
Figure 3-142

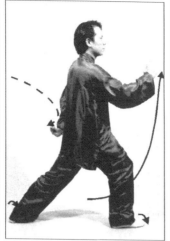
Figure 3-143

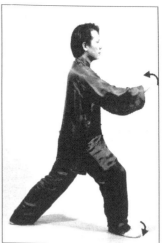
Figure 3-144

Posture 17: Lower Body Then Stand on One Leg - Right

Movements: (Figures 3-140 to 3-145)

Step 1. Put the ball of your right foot down in front of you. At the same time raise your left hand up and change it into a hook, and bring your right hand next to your left shoulder, palm in (Figure 3-140).

Shift some weight onto your right foot, and turn your left foot out. Then shift all your weight back to your left foot (Figure 3-141).

Step 2. Step West with your right foot, as you lower your right hand towards your right foot (Figure 3-142).

Step 3. Shift your weight forward into a right Bow Stance, as you turn your front foot forward and back foot in. At the same time, extend your right hand forward then up in front of you, and lower your left hand down and rotate the hook to point up (Figure 3-143).

Step 4. Turn your right foot out slightly as you rotate your right hand so your palm faces down (Figure 3-144).

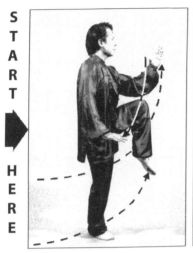

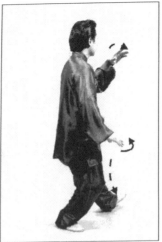

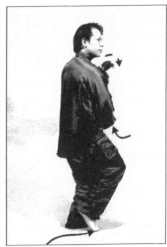

Figure 3-145   Figure 3-146   Figure 3-147

Shift all your weight forward onto your right foot and stand up, with your left knee as high as you can. At the same time, brush your right hand down to the side of your hip, with your palm facing down; then open your left hand and lift it up to eye level in front of you, with your palm facing to the right (Figure 3-145).

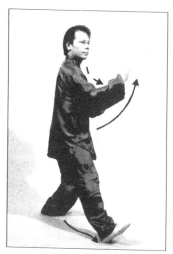
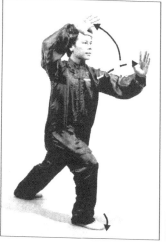
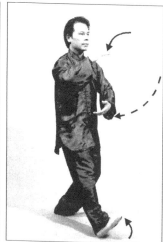

Figure 3-148   Figure 3-149   Figure 3-150

Posture 18: Shuttle Back and Forth

Movements: (Figures 3-146 to 3-153)

Step 1. *Right*: Lower your body by bending your right knee. Turn your body and step Southwest with your left foot (Figure 3-146).

Shift all your weight onto your left foot and bring your right foot next to your left. At the same time, hold the Taiji Ball in front of your chest, left hand up, right hand down (Figure 3-147).

Step 2. Step Northwest with your right foot and shift your weight forward into a right Bow Stance. At the same time, raise your right arm to the upper right corner and extend your left hand forward (Figures 3-148 and 3-149).

Step 3. *Left*: Shift your weight back to your left foot and lower your arms down into a holding the Taiji Ball position, right hand up, left hand down (Figure 3-150).

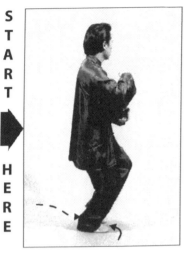
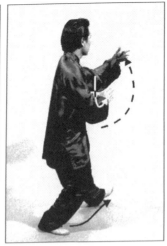
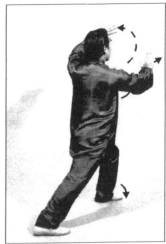

Figure 3-151   Figure 3-152   Figure 3-153

Turn your right foot out slightly. Shift all your weight on to your right foot and bring your left foot next to your right foot (Figure 3-151).

Step 4. Step Southwest with your left foot and shift your weight forward into a left Bow Stance. At the same time, raise your left arm to the upper left corner and extend your right hand forward (Figures 3-152 and 3-153).

Note:

1. Shuttle Back and Forth is referring to a weaver's shuttle, moving back and forth.

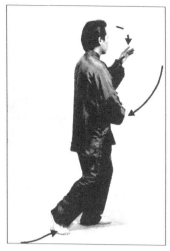

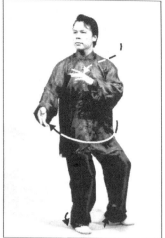

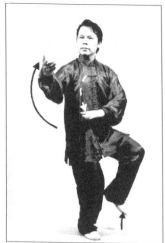

| Figure 3-154 | Figure 3-155 | Figure 3-156 |

Posture 19: Needle at Sea Bottom

Movements: (Figures 3-154 to 3-157)

Step 1. Shift all your weight forward as you bring your right foot behind your left foot; and begin lowering your arms (Figure 3-154). Shift all your weight back to your right foot. Turn your body towards your right (Figure 3-155).

Step 2. Brush your left hand across your body and down next to your left hip; and raise your right hand up to eye level then spear down and forward in front of you. At the same time, raise your left foot off the floor and touch down on the ball of your foot in front of you (Figures 3-156 and 3-157).

Notes:

1. When standing in an Empty stance (with all the weight on one leg), only go as low as you can without putting undue strain on your knee.

2. Keep your right knee pointing in the same direction as your right foot to prevent unnecessary torsion on your knee.

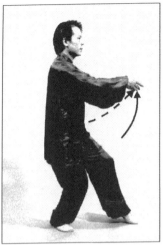

Figure 3-157 Figure 3-158 Figure 3-159

Posture 20: Fan Through Back

Movements: (Figures 3-158 to 3-160)

Step 1. Bring your left hand next to your right wrist and lift both arms up. At the same time, step forward with your left foot into a left Bow Stance (Figures 3-158 and 3-159).

Step 2. Turn your body slightly toward your right as you lift your right arm up, palm out, and extend your left hand forward, palm forward (Figure 3-160).

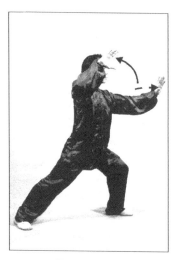

Figure 3-160

Note:

1. The Chinese name for this posture is Shantongbei. *Shan* means fan. In the posture the hands move apart and the arms are extended resembling a Chinese fan. *Tongbei* means through the back. It implies that the movement/power is emitted by passing through your back (spine) and out to your arms.

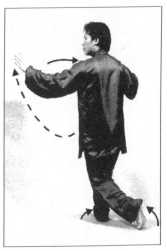 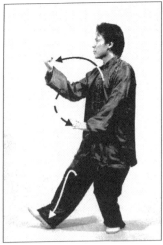 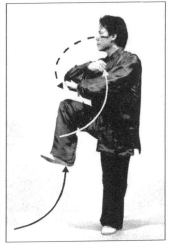

Figure 3-166   Figure 3-165   Figure 3-164

Posture 21: Turn Body, Deflect, Parry, and Punch

Movements: (Figures 3-161 to 3-168)

Step 1. Turn your body around 180 degrees by shifting your weight back, turning your left foot in and right foot out. At the same time, extend your right arm towards your right (Figures 3-161 and 3-162).

Step 2. Shift your weight back to your left foot. At the same time, change your right hand into a fist and circle down; bend your left elbow and begin lowering your left hand (Figure 3-163).

Step 3. Shift all your weight back to your left foot. Lift your right foot up and touch down with your heel, in front of you. At the same time, continue to lower your left hand down to your waist level, and circle your right fist in, then forward (Figures 3-164 and 3-165).

Step 4. Turn your right foot out while stepping forward with your left foot. At the same time, circle your right fist to your right, then down next to your waist; and lower your left hand slightly, then up in front of your body (Figures 3-166 and 3-167).

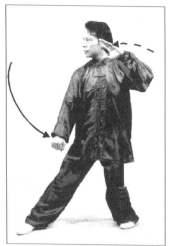

Figure 3-163

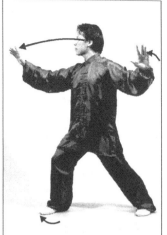

Figure 3-162

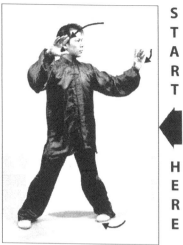

Figure 3-161

S
T
A
R
T

H
E
R
E

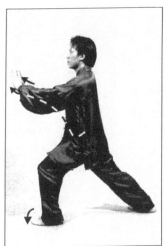
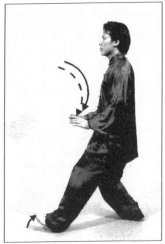
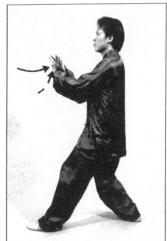

Figure 3-172   Figure 3-171   Figure 3-170

Step 5. Shift your weight forward into a left Bow Stance. At the same time, punch forward with your right fist. Finish with your left hand gently touching the inside of your right forearm (Figure 3-168).

Note:

1. As you circle your right fist in and out, also lift your right foot up and down. Imagine that your hand is like the crank shaft of a train wheel, rotating the wheel (right foot) in a circular motion.

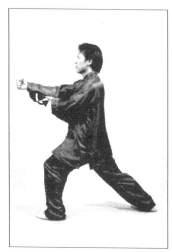
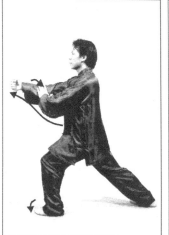
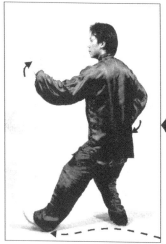

S
T
A
R
T

H
E
R
E

Figure 3-169   Figure 3-168   Figure 3-167

Posture 22: Seal Tightly and Follow with a Push

Movements: (Figures 3-169 to 3-172)

Step 1. Maintain contact with your left hand and your right forearm, while rotating your left palm to the outside of your right elbow (Figure 3-169).

Shift your weight back to your right foot and rotate both palms to face in as you slide your left hand up your right forearm. (Figure 3-170). Separate and lower both hands down next to your abdomen and lift the ball of your left foot up. (Figure 3-171).

Step 2. Put your left foot down and shift your weight forward, back into a left Bow Stance. At the same time, push forward with your hands (Figures 3-172).

Note:

1. The push movement resembles the push movement in the Grasp the Sparrow's Tail posture.

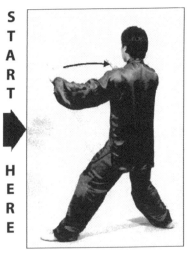
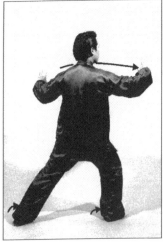
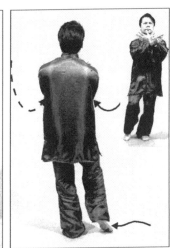

Figure 3-173	Figure 3-174	Figure 3-175

Posture 23: Cross Hands

Movements: (Figures 3-173 to 3-176)

Step 1. Turn your body around 180 degrees as you turn your left foot in and right foot out while shifting your weight towards your right foot. At the same time, extend your right arm towards your right (Figures 3-173 and 3-174).

Step 2. Shift all your weight back to your left foot, bring your right foot next to your left, then step out again a shoulder width apart. At the same time, lower your hands then cross your arms in front of your chest. (Figures 3-175 and 3-176, Face South).

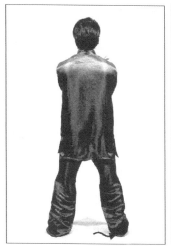
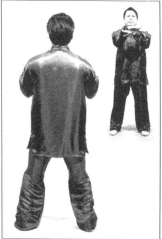
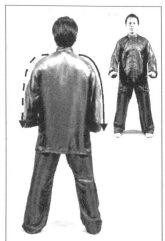

Figure 3-176   Figure 3-177   Figure 3-178

Posture 24: Closing

Movements: (Figures 3-177 to 3-179)

Step 1. Rotate both hands until your palms are facing down (Figure 3-177).

Step 2. Separate your hands to shoulder width apart. Then lower both hands, palms down, to hip level and stand up completely. (Figure 3-178). Bring your left foot next to your right and relax hands down to your sides (Figure 3-179).

Note:

1. At the end, pause or casually walk for a few minutes, to feel the flow of qi throughout your entire body; allowing the qi to redistribute, balance, repair, and strengthen your entire body.

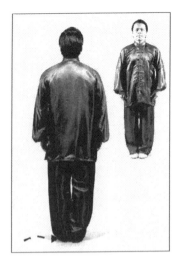

Figure 3-179

Appendix: Lesson Plan

Like everything else we do, a well-planned course of action and dedicated determination are required to achieve the best possible success. Learning Taijiquan (Tai Chi Chuan) also requires planning, action, and follow through with a plan. In the pages that follow we have laid out the learning of this routine into 12 Lessons. Work on each lesson until you are comfortable with the movements. You may wish to spend a few days to a week or more on each lesson before continuing with the next lesson.

In Chinese, there is a term known as "gongfu". It is an attainment, whether it be attaining better health, healing, proficiency in painting or cooking. Gongfu attainment requires that the participant actively engage in working and experiencing the specific task at hand. Now that you have made a commitment to studying and practicing Taijiquan, it is important that you set aside some time each week for the learning and practicing of Taijiquan.

Set aside 1/2 hour to 1 hour, 3 to 7 days a week. Learn one section of the routine at a time. Repeat as many times and days as necessary so that you will not forget the movements. You may wish to work on the upper body and the legs separately before combining the movements.

Today we have tools that help us achieve our goals much faster and efficiently than ever before. This book is designed so that you may be able to learn from it without a teacher, however, we strongly advise that you have the guidance of a properly trained professional Taijiquan Instructor. This book is the right tool for beginners to learn the Simplified (24) Posture Taijiquan. To learn other Taijiquan routines other tools may be necessary. You may also wish to obtain a videotape of this routine as an additional reference and learning tool.

Lesson Plan

Lesson 1

1. Read Chapter 1 and Chapter 2 of this book.

2. Recognize and warm up the 9 joint group areas.

3. Learn to move your spine.

4. Learn the Taiji Qigong method.

    Write down some of your insights and notes for yourself, or write down some questions for your instructor.

Lesson 2

1. Learn the Preparation.

2. Learn Posture 1: Taiji Beginning 起势

3. Learn Posture 2: Part the Wild Horse's Mane 左右野馬分鬃

    Write down some of your insights and notes for yourself, or write down some questions for your instructor.

Lesson 3

1. Learn Posture 3: White Crane Spreads Its Wings 白鶴亮翅

2. Learn Posture 4: Brush Knee and Step Forward 左右摟膝拗步
   Write down some of your insights and notes for yourself,
   or write down some questions for your instructor.

Lesson 4

1. Learn Posture 5: Playing the Lute 手揮琵琶

2. Learn Posture 6: Repulse Monkey 左右倒攆猴
   Write down some of your insights and notes for yourself,
   or write down some questions for your instructor.

Lesson 5

1. Learn Posture 7: Grasp Sparrow's Tail - Left 左攬雀尾
     Write down some of your insights and notes for yourself, or write down some questions for your instructor.

Lesson 6

1. Learn Posture 8: Grasp Sparrow's Tail - Right 右攬雀尾
     Write down some of your insights and notes for yourself, or write down some questions for your instructor.

Lesson 7

1. Learn Posture 9: Single Whip 單鞭

2. Learn Posture 10: Wave Hands Like Clouds 雲手

3. Learn Posture 11: Single Whip 單鞭

    Write down some of your insights and notes for yourself, or write down some questions for your instructor.

Lesson 8

1. Learn Posture 12: High Pat on Horse 高探馬

2. Learn Posture 13: Right Heel Kick 右蹬腳

3. Learn Posture 14: Strike to Ears with Both Fists 雙峰貫耳

    Write down some of your insights and notes for yourself, or write down some questions for your instructor.

Lesson 9

1. Learn Posture 15: Turn Body and Left Heel Kick 轉身左蹬腳

2. Learn Posture 16: Lower Body and Stand on One Leg - Left
   左下勢獨立
   Write down some of your insights and notes for yourself,
   or write down some questions for your instructor.

Lesson 10

1. Learn Posture 17: Lower Body and Stand on One Leg - Right
   右下勢獨立
   Write down some of your insights and notes for yourself,
   or write down some questions for your instructor.

Lesson 11

1. Learn Posture 18: Shuttle Back and Forth 左右穿梭

2. Learn Posture 19: Needle at Sea Bottom 海底針

3. Learn Posture 20: Fan Through Back 閃通背

   Write down some of your insights and notes for yourself, or write down some questions for your instructor.

Lesson 12

1. Learn Posture 21: Turn Body, Deflect, Parry, and Punch 轉身搬攔捶

2. Learn Posture 22: Seal Tightly and Follow with a Push 如封似閉

3. Learn Posture 23: Cross Hands 十字手

4. Learn Posture 24: Closing 收勢

   Write down some of your insights and notes for yourself, or write down some questions for your instructor.

Bibliography

1. Liang, Shou-Yu & Wu, Wen-Ching. *Qigong Empowerment: A Guide to Medical, Taoist, Buddhist, and Wushu Energy Cultivation.* Rhode Island, The Way of the Dragon Publishing, 1997.

About the Author:

Master Wu, Wen-Ching

Master Wu is an international expert, and a gifted practitioner and teacher of Tai Chi, Qigong and Chinese martial arts. His primary teachers and mentors are Grandmaster Liang, Shouyu, Professor Wang, Jurong, and Dr. Wu, Chengde. In 1990 he ended his engineering career and dedicated himself into learning, preserving and teaching the empowering techniques of these ancient arts. Since then, he has published many authoritative books on the subjects and received many honors and awards:

Honors and Awards:
- China's Contemporary Wushu Master
- Top Ten Wushu Coach of the World
- Top 100 Wushu Extraordinare
- World Renowned Martial Artist
- Sanshoudao 8th Level Black Belt Master Instructor
- Two All-Around Champion Awards-US Wushu National
- Three Gold Medals-Shanghai, China International Wushu Festival
- BS Mechanical Engineering Northeastern University, Boston MA

Publications:
- *Qigong Empowerments*
- *Kung Fu Elements*
- *Tai Chi Beginning*
- *Simplified Taijiquan*
- *Tai Chi Single Fan*
- *Sword Imperatives*
- *Xiaoyaoshuai*
- *Emei Baguazhang*

School and publications for Health, Healing, and Martial Arts

The Way of the Dragon was founded in Rhode Island by Master Wu, Wen-Ching in 1990. Over the past two decades the school has established itself as one of the most authoritative centers of its kind in the U.S. The Way of the Dragon offers comprehensive programs and publications to assist practitioners in their health, healing, and martial arts pursuits.

Our programs include classes to empower students from a tender age of 3 to 100 years young! Master Wu's vision of creating a positive environment to which students are encouraged to take an active role in their personal health and well-being, has been realized by thousands of participants. Today, at his East Providence school, Master Wu and instructors personally taught by him continue to provide the highest quality of instruction to participant from all-over New England. Master Wu also provides in-house and on-site workshops in the U.S. and worldwide, as well as, provide individual lessons and corporate consultations. Below are some of the topics of his classes and workshops:

Health and Healing Classes
- Tai Chi
- Medical Qigong
- Taoist Qigong
- Buddhist Qigong
- Emitting and Absorbing Qigong

Internal & External Martial Arts Classes
- Emei Shaolin Kung Fu
- Contemporary Wushu
- Tai Chi Chuan
- Xingyiquan
- Baguazhang
- Liuhebafa
- Hard Qigong

Index

Printed in Great Britain
by Amazon